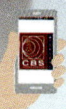

Orthopaedic Clinics

HIP

With Video Demonstration

Copy of the Review

Indian J Orthop. 2008 Apr-Jun; 42(2): 238.

ORTHOPAEDIC CLINICS: SPINE

**Sudhir K Kapoor. CBS Publishers and Distributors, New Delhi
ISBN: 978-81-239-1599-9.**

What I like about this book is that it is a good tool to learn about the examination of the spine for the residents and it serves as a quick reference on his way to examining a patient with spinal disease and disorder. The book is easy to read and each chapter is well elaborated with abundant illustrations, figures and drawings. It also has a chapter on "How to infer examination findings", which gives a comprehensive method to diagnose a particular injury or disease of the spine, which may have evolved over a period of time. There is an added advantage of a video format, which facilitates learning for the medical students and the residents. In my opinion, the book is useful and of great help to the residents in strengthening their concept in clinical methods and improving the quality of case presentation. I recommend this book for the medical students and the trainees at all levels and also to the general practitioners who treat patients with spinal problems and may then refer these patients to an orthopaedic surgeon.

The Four-Volume Series

Orthopaedic Clinics

SPINE

HIP

KNEE

SHOULDER AND ELBOW

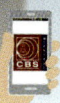

Orthopaedic Clinics

HIP

With Video Demonstration

Sudhir K Kapoor

MS (Orthopaedics), FRCS (Glasgow)

Professor, Department of Orthopaedics
SGT Medical College and Hospital
Budhera, Gurugram, Haryana

Former
Head, Department of Orthopaedics and Chief of Ortho-oncology
Indian Spinal Injuries Centre, New Delhi

Professor and Head, Department of Orthopaedics
Lady Hardinge Medical College and Associated Hospitals, New Delhi
Dean, ESI PGIMSR, New Delhi

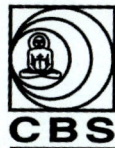

CBS

CBS Publishers & Distributors Pvt Ltd

New Delhi • Bengaluru • Chennai • Kochi • Kolkata • Mumbai
Bhopal • Bhubaneswar • Hyderabad • Jharkhand • Nagpur
Patna • Pune • Uttarakhand • Dhaka (Bangladesh) • Kathmandu (Nepal)

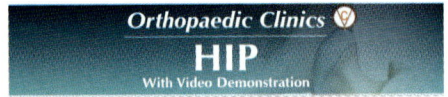

ISBN: 978-93-89261-81-3

First Edition: 2020

Published by Satish Kumar Jain and produced by Varun Jain for

CBS Publishers & Distributors Pvt Ltd

4819/XI Prahlad Street, 24 Ansari Road, Daryaganj, New Delhi 110 002, India.
Ph: 23289259, 23266861, 23266867   Fax: 011-23243014
Website: www.cbspd.com   e-mail: delhi@cbspd.com; cbspubs@airtelmail.in.

Corporate Office: 204 FIE, Industrial Area, Patparganj, Delhi 110 092, India
Ph: 4934 4934   Fax: 4934 4935   e-mail: publishing@cbspd.com; publicity@cbspd.com

Branches

- **Bengaluru:** Seema House 2975, 17th Cross, K.R. Road, Banasankari 2nd Stage, Bengaluru 560 070, Karnataka, India
  Ph: +91-80-26771678/79   Fax: +91-80-26771680   e-mail: bangalore@cbspd.com
- **Chennai:** 7, Subbaraya Street, Shenoy Nagar, Chennai 600 030, Tamil Nadu, India.
  Ph: +91-44-26680620, 26681266   Fax: +91-44-42032115   e-mail: chennai@cbspd.com
- **Kochi:** 68/1534, 35, 36 Power House Road, Opposite KSEB, Kochi-682018, Kerala, India.
  Ph: +91-484-4059061-65   Fax: +91-484-4059065   e-mail: kochi@cbspd.com
- **Kolkata:** 6/B, Ground Floor, Rameswar Shaw Road, Kolkata-700 014 (West Bengal), India.
  Ph: +91-33-2289-1126, 2289-1127, 2289-1128   e-mail: kolkata@cbspd.com
- **Mumbai:** 83-C, Dr E Moses Road, Worli, Mumbai-400018, Maharashtra, India.
  Ph: +91-22-24902340/41   Fax: +91-22-24902342   e-mail: mumbai@cbspd.com

Representatives

- **Bhopal**   0-8319310552
- **Jharkhand**   0-9811541605
- **Pune**   0-9623451994
- **Dhaka (Bangladesh)** 01912-003485
- **Bhubaneswar**   0-9911037372
- **Nagpur**   0-9421945513
- **Uttarakhand**   0-9716462459
- **Kathmandu (Nepal)** 977-9818742655
- **Hyderabad**   0-9885175004
- **Patna**   0-9334159340

Printed at: Nutech Print Services, Faridabad, India

to

My parents

Ram Lal and Sudershan Kapoor
(with blessings from heaven)

Wife Suma

Children Saurabh & Parminder and Sudeep & Shaweta

and

My patients

Foreword

It is indeed my pleasure to pen my words as a foreword for the new book on hip examination, authored by Dr Sudhir K Kapoor, who is a senior and respected professor, and a seasoned examiner. Going through the pages, his tenacity of purpose and will to help the students, the registrars and the consultants alike in making the hip examination easier, is obvious. Hip examination is like a mathematical derivation, and each of the chapters from anatomy to the radiological interpretation has been laid out sequentially, and well illustrated.

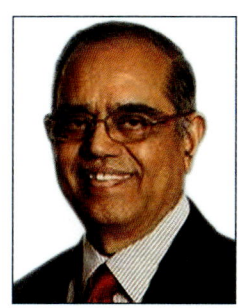

In a recent CME Program in Kolkata, a German surgeon asked me a relevant question after my presentation of hip examination, as to whether it is necessary to go into such details in examination, when the investigations specially imaging studies can give an immediate picture. I replied him that 10% of spine cases are wrongly operated without an examination of hip; and 10% of hips are wrongly operated without a proper clinical examination of spine and the ipsilateral knee. Moreover, patients vocation, his habits and his requirements, which will become apparent after a through clinical history and examination, will help to decide the best suited management of that particular patient.

Just like his previous illustrated book on examination of the spine, this book, I am sure, will be a handbook to all of us.

May God bless this work and him in all his endeavours.

Prof (Dr) M Shantharam Shetty
MS (Ortho), FICS (Ortho), FIAMS
Director, Tejasvini Hospital, Mangalore

Preface

Since the time my first book *Orthopaedic Clinics: Spine* was published about 9 years ago, there has been an exponential increase in the number of postgraduate education courses in many parts of India, several of which I have participated. I have been instrumental in stimulating this growth of PG courses, and I utilized my tenure in Indian Orthopaedic Association to further this cause.

These courses have successfully enhanced the level of knowledge and skill in postgraduate students appearing for their certificate exams. I am able to gauge this improvement, since I have been involved in PG training for more than 30 years. However, a lot has still to be achieved in this field of postgraduate training in our country. My work on clinical examination of hip is an effort in this direction.

The language and the information in this book have been deliberately kept basic, with plenty of diagrams and illustrations, to make the subject clear. The hallmark of this venture is the associated presentation on the App, which can be accessed by the person who purchases this book. The presentation contains the different clinical signs, demonstrated on the real patients (not volunteers). These patients have been seen and the cases collected over a period of many years of my working in different medical colleges of Delhi.

This work is not a replacement for bedside examination, which remains indispensible to really learn the art of patient examination. I still like to again stress the quote from my previous book on spine examination—the patient is the "best teacher" and the teacher is a mere guide to direct pupil in the right direction. To take maximum benefit from the book, the student must read it first, see my presentation on the net and then apply the same to his patient immediately, keeping this book as a handy guide, if any doubt arises.

I will strongly recommend that the examinee follows a definite sequence of clinical examination of the hip, which is to be repeated in the same sequence, maximum number of times. It will ensure that the examinee does not miss any sign, either during the examination, or in his clinical practice in his later life, after he is board qualified.

Happy Learning!

Sudhir K Kapoor

Acknowledgements

I am extremely thankful to all the colleagues, both junior and senior, in the Department of Orthopaedic Surgery, Lady Harding Medical College and ESI PGIMSR, New Delhi, who have helped in this project.

The help from a few colleagues have been very substantial. I specially appreciate the help from Dr Harsimar Singh, postgraduate resident, who has been very patient in editing and improving the final draft. Dr Sandeep Singh, senior resident, was always forthcoming in giving the shape to the text and editing videos. I fondly remember, many Sundays and holidays when I sat together with Dr Harsimar Singh and Dr Sandeep Singh to complete the project, particularly in the later stages. Dr Anjul, PG resident was another colleague very helpful for finalizing the video demonstration of a few orthopaedic tests.

The basic format of the accompanying video presentation was prepared by Dr Siddharth, my resident in Lady Harding Medical College. I am thankful to him.

I am thankful to my publishers, particularly Mr. YN Arjuna (Senior Vice-President, Publishing, Editorial and Publicity), for bringing out an excellent presentation.

In the end, I am really obliged to all my patients, who willingly and ungrudgingly helped to complete the visual input of accompanying presentation.

Sudhir K Kapoor

Reviews and Comments

The *Orthopaedic Clinics: HIP* is the 2nd book by the author. His 1st book is extremely popular with the PG students. On the persuasion of his colleagues, Dr Kapoor has written the 2nd book for the PG students. Eliciting the clinical signs is very important from examination point of view. This has been very explicitly given in the book. The beauty of the book is that it has many good illustrations and photographs which are very helpful in understanding the point. The relevant anatomy and the gait analysis have been beautifully described before going to the clinical part. The biomechanics of the hip joint has been explained in a very simple manner.

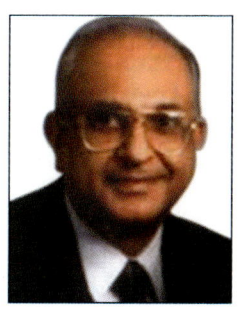

I am confident that this book will prove a boon to all orthopaedic trainees, because in the exit examination, 70% students get hip examination. They are asked to demonstrate the physical signs and very often they get confused because they are not clear about the clinical tests. This book is going to fill this void.

I strongly recommend the *Orthopaedic Clinics: HIP* written by Dr Sudhir K Kapoor to all orthopaedic trainees and this book must find a place on the shelf of each and every library.

Dr DK Taneja
D.orth, MS (orth), FAMS, FRCS (Eng), FIOA
Prof and HOD of Orthopaedic and Medical Director,
Arihant Hospital and Research Centre, Indore
DNB Coordinator
Founder Director, MGM Allied Health Sciences Institute (MAHSI)
Chairman CME Committee, NAMS
President World Orthopaedic Concern
Secretary Orthopaedic Research and Education Foundation, India
Past President, Orthopaedic Association of SAARC Countries
Past President, Indian Orthopaedic Association
Emeritus Prof, Sri Aurbindo Institute of Medical Sciences, Indore
Director, Centre for Science and Society, Indore
Ex-Dean, MGM Medical College, Indore

*O*rthopaedic Clinics: HIP is an essential book for postgraduate trainees. It can also be a good reference for undergraduate students when they wish to understand clinical examination in detail; and to junior consultants, sitting in the OPD, the accompanying presentation in which all the clinical signs have been demonstrated on the patients is the most important aspect of this book. The language of the book is very precise and principles have been explained well, which can be understood and retained easily by the students. The book has a lot of illustrations collected over decades to make the subject interesting. The nine chapters 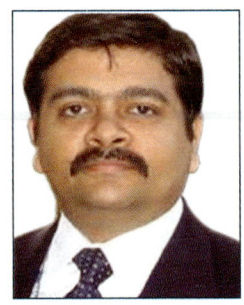 in this book are very complete and relevant in a desired sequence. A special mention is about the chapter on gait. Being a difficult topic, it has not been covered in any book the way a student needs it. Each part of clinical examination being addressed as a chapter is a very good concept emphasizing the importance of each. Interpreting findings of clinical examination is an aspect which one learns with time, it is nice to see that interpretation is also a complete chapter. In all, this is an excellent gift from our beloved Dr Sudhir K Kapoor sir to the budding orthopaedic surgeons of tomorrow.

Dr Lalit Maini
MS, (Orthopaedics)
Director Professor
Maulana Azad Medical College,
New Delhi

*T*his book by eminent author and excellent teacher, Dr Sudhir K Kapoor is very informative and incredibly refreshing. The methodical demonstration of various signs in the accompanying presentation makes it an indispensable guide. Its analytical approach through individual chapters with rich illustrations makes it a highly valuable resource for postgraduate students and young consultants 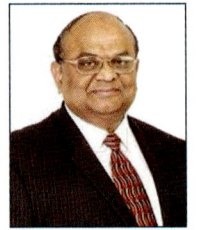 starting the career. I thoroughly recommend it.

Dr Mayil Vahanan Natarajan
MS (Orth), MCh (Orth)(L'pool),
PhD (Orth Onco), FRCS (Eng)

Contents

Relevant Anatomy of Hip

+ Components of hip joint
+ Capsule and ligaments of hip joint
+ Muscle groups around the hip joint
+ Trabecular pattern of the hip

+ Angular orientation of upper end of femur and acetabulum
+ Biomechanical factors working around the hip
+ Blood supply of femoral head

COMPONENTS OF HIP JOINT

Articulation of the head of the femur with the acetabulum of the pelvic bone is a ball and socket variety of synovial joint (Fig. 1.1). This typical ball and socket offers unusually good mobility, like the movement of circumduction which is not present in any other joint of the lower limb. This tremendous mobility is at the cost of some amount of stability, i.e. the possibility of dislocation increases. This compromised stability is to some extent, compensated by the hip joint capsule with its unusually strong ligaments and a fibrocartilaginous ring all along the margin of acetabulum. This fibrocartilaginous ring is called acetabular labrum, which deepens the cavity of the acetabular fossa (Figs 1.2 and 1.3).

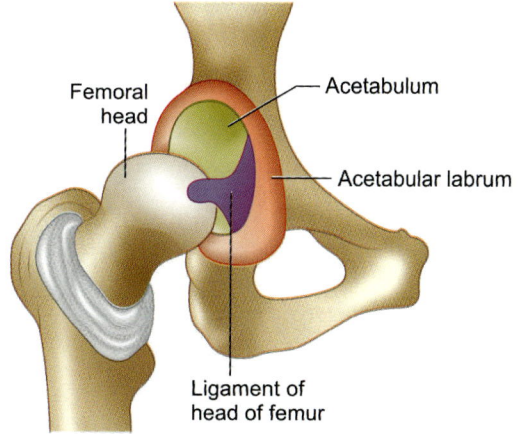
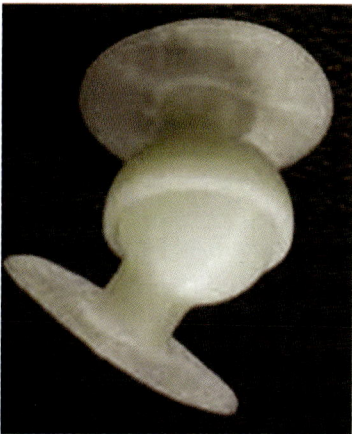

Fig. 1.1: Hip joint—ball and socket type

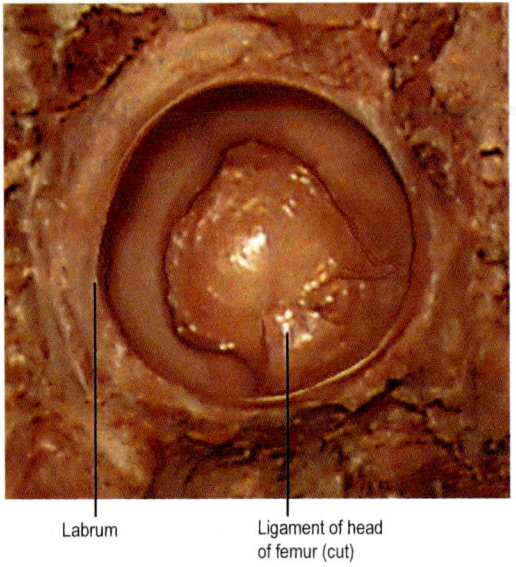

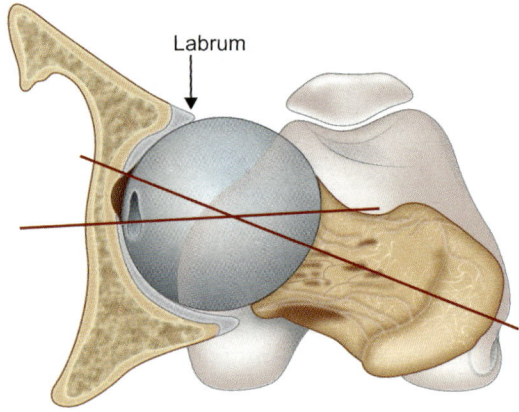

Fig. 1.2: Capsule and labrum of acetabulum

Fig. 1.3: Labrum—makes the acetabular cavity deep

The hip joint serves the important purpose of transmitting the body weight through the sacroiliac joint to the lower limb (Fig. 1.4).

CAPSULE AND LIGAMENTS OF HIP JOINT

Capsule of the hip joint is attached proximally to the rim of acetabulum. Distally, it is attached anteriorly to intertrochanteric line, and posteriorly to the neck of femur, about ½ inch proximal to the intertrochanteric crest. The anterior attachment of the capsule at the intertrochanteric line is quite firm while attachment to the posterior aspect of the neck is weak.

This anatomical fact of the shorter extent of posterior part of capsule in comparison to the anterior part has a clinical relevance. Intertrochanteric fractures are mostly extra-articular and, therefore, lead to an exaggerated external rotation deformity of the ipsilateral lower limb, since the restraining force of capsule is absent (Fig. 1.5). In comparison, basicervical fractures are partly intra-articular and other neck fractures are completely intra-articular. It leads to the restraining force of hip capsule to come into play and the amount of external rotation of the lower limb is restricted (Fig. 1.6), compared to intertrochanteric fractures.

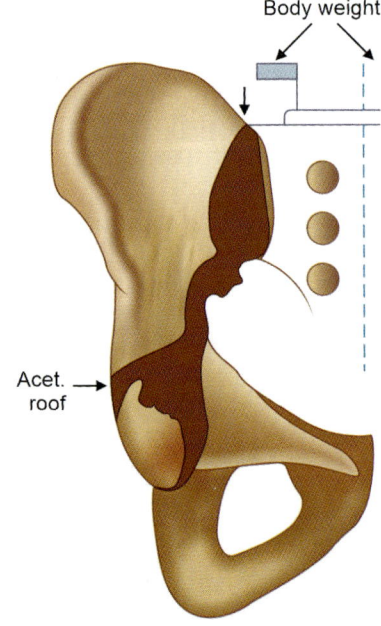

Fig. 1.4: Weight transmission axis from sacrum to acetabular roof

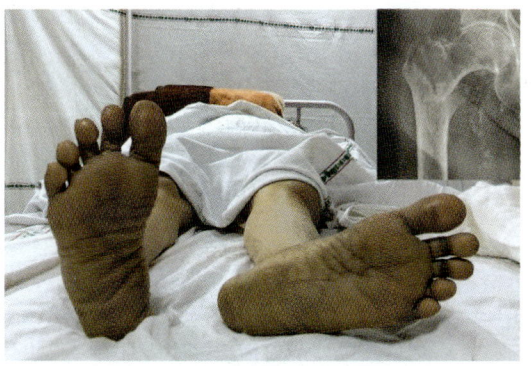 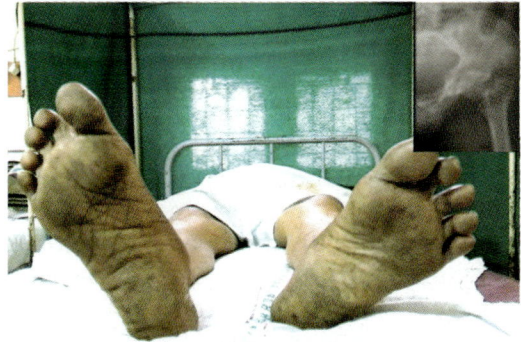

Fig. 1.5: Intertrochanteric fracture, gross external rotation of the foot (lateral border of foot touching the bed)

Fig. 1.6: Intracapsular neck of femur fracture, external rotation less than intertrochanteric fracture

There are three ligaments which strengthen the capsule and are infact blended with the capsule.

1. **Iliofemoral ligament or the ligament of Bigelow** (Fig. 1.7): It is the thickest and the strongest, and is located anteriorly. It is shaped like an inverted Y. It arises from the anterior inferior iliac spine and the adjacent rim of the acetabulum. It then spreads obliquely downwards and laterally to divide into two limbs which are attached to the intertrochanteric line, giving it the appearance of an inverted Y. This ligament is tightened when hip is extended and is the chief stabilizer of hip joint in erect position

2. **Pubofemoral ligament** (Fig. 1.7): It is present on inferior aspect of the hip joint. This ligament is attached, superiorly to the obturator crest and the superior ramus of the pubis; inferiorly, it blends with the capsule and with the deep surface of the vertical band of the iliofemoral ligament.

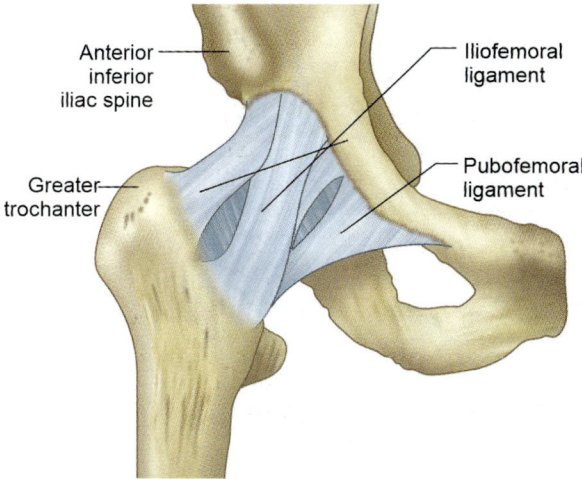 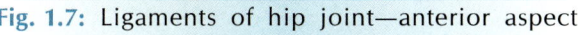 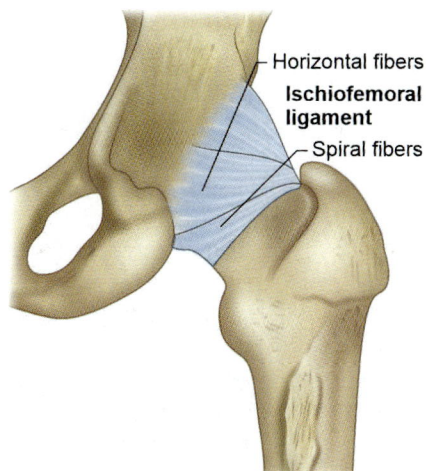

Fig. 1.7: Ligaments of hip joint—anterior aspect

Fig. 1.8: Ligaments of the hip joint—posterior aspect

3. **Ischiofemoral ligament** (Fig. 1.8)**:** It is present posteriorly. Its fibers span from the ischium, at a point below and behind the acetabulum, to blend with the circular fibers at the posterior end of the joint capsule. Through the posterior capsule, it gains attachment at the posterior aspect of neck of femur, ¼ inch proximal to intertrochanteric line.

These ligaments are very strong and disruption of these ligaments indicates severe injury as happens in hip dislocation. Even in instances of hip dislocation, the strongest of the three, the iliofemoral ligament usually escapes injury. The intact iliofemoral ligament along with the spasm of iliopsoas muscle in cases of posterior dislocation of hip is responsible for typical adduction, flexion and internal rotation deformity of the ipsilateral lower limb. In those rare cases of posterior dislocation of the hip joint, where iliofemoral ligament is also disrupted, the typical deformity of flexion, adduction, and internal rotation is absent. This is called 'irregular hip dislocation'.

Transverse Ligament of Acetabulum

The circle of the acetabular ring, deficient in its inferior part, is completed by a transverse ligament—transverse acetabular ligament (TAL) (Fig. 1.9). This ligament has a significant role in hip surgery. It serves as a guide for the correct placement of acetabular component of the total hip prosthesis (particularly anteversion and inclination). Transverse acetabular ligament remains intact, even in cases of advanced hip disease, and is helpful anatomical structure for reference during hip replacement surgery.

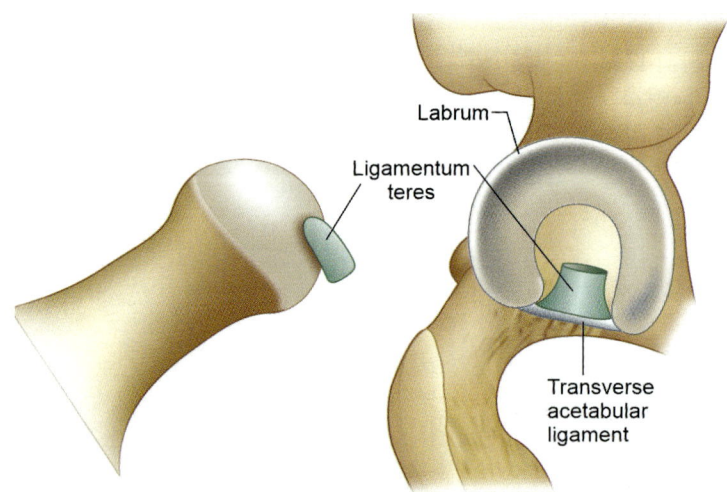

Fig. 1.9: Transverse acetabular ligament

MUSCLE GROUPS AROUND THE HIP JOINT

Flexors of Hip (Table 1.1)

Flexors of the hip are:
- Iliopsoas (iliacus and psoas major)
- Rectus femoris (part of quadriceps femoris)

Table 1.1: Flexors of hip joint

Name	Proximal attachment	Distal attachment	Innervation	Action	
Iliacus	Iliac fossa	Base of lesser trochanter	Femoral nerve (L2, L3, L4)	Flexion of hip	
Psoas major	Transverse processes of T12 to L5	Lesser trochanter	Anterior rami of L1, L2, L3 nerves	Flexion of hip	
Rectus femoris	Straight head from upper half of anterior inferior spine; Reflected head from groove above acetabulum	Quadriceps tendon	Femoral nerve (L2, L3, L4)	Extension of knee; assists in flexion of hip	

Extensors of Hip

Extensors of the hip are (Table 1.2):
- Gluteus maximus
- Hamstrings muscle group (biceps femoris, semimembranosus, semitendinosus)

Table 1.2: Extensors of hip joint

Name	Proximal attachment	Distal attachment	Innervation	Action	
Gluteus maximus	Gluteal surface of ilium, lumbar fascia, sacrum, sacrotuberous ligament	Deep part in gluteal tuberosity of femur; and superficial part in iliotibial tract	Inferior gluteal nerve (L5, S1, S2)	External rotation and extension of the hip joint, and helps extension of knee through iliotibial tract	
Biceps femoris	Long head from ischial tuberosity; Short head from linea aspera	Head of fibula	Long head— tibial nerve; Short head— common fibular nerve	Extension of hip and flexion of knee	
Semi-membranosus	Lateral part of ischial tuberosity	Medial condyle of tibia	Tibial part of sciatic nerve (L5, S1, S2)	Extension of hip and flexion of knee	
Semitendi-nosus	Medial part of ischial tuberosity	Upper part of medial surface of tibia	Tibial part of sciatic nerve (L5, S1, S2)	Extension of hip and flexion of knee	

Adductors of Hip

Muscles causing adduction at the hip joint are (Table 1.3):

- Adductor longus
- Adductor brevis
- Adductor magnus
- Gracilis
- Pectineus

Name	Proximal attachment	Distal attachment	Innervation	Action	
Table 1.3: Adductors of hip joint					
Adductor longus	Pubic body, between pubic crest and symphysis	Middle third of the linea aspera of femur	Anterior division of obturator nerve (L2, L3, L4)	Adduction of hip, flexion of hip	
Adductor brevis	Body and inferior ramus of pubic bone	Linea aspera and lesser trochanter	Anterior division of obturator nerve (L2, L3, L4)	Adduction of hip	
Adductor magnus (formed by fusion of adductor and hamstring muscle masses)	Hamstring part from ischial tuberosity, adductor part from ischiopubic ramus	Hamstring part to adductor tubercle, adductor part to linea aspera	Hamstring part by tibial part of sciatic nerve, adductor part by posterior division of obturator nerve	Adduction of hip is the primary action Hamstring part assists in extension of hip Adductor part assists in flexion of hip	

Contd.

Table 1.3: Adductors of hip joint (*Contd.*)

Name	Proximal attachment	Distal attachment	Innervation	Action	
Gracilis	Ischiopubic ramus	Upper part of medial surface of tibia	Anterior division of obturator nerve (L2, L3, L4)	Adduction, flexion and medial rotation of hip	
Pectineus	Pectineal line of pubis	Pectineal line, below lesser trochanter	Anterior division of femoral nerve (L2–L4)	Adduction and flexion of hip	

Abductors of Hip

Muscles causing abduction at the hip joint are (Table 1.4):
- Gluteus medius
- Gluteus minimus

Table 1.4: Abductors of hip joint

Name	Proximal attachment	Distal attachment	Innervation	Action	
Gluteus medius	Gluteal surface of ilium between middle and posterior gluteal lines	Greater trochanter	Superior gluteal nerve (L4, L5, S1)	Abduction of hip	

Contd.

Table 1.4: Abductors of hip joint (Contd.)					
Name	**Proximal Attachment**	**Distal Attachment**	**Innervation**	**Action**	
Gluteus minimus	Gluteal surface of ilium between middle and inferior gluteal lines	Greater trochanter	Superior gluteal nerve (L4, L5, S1)	Abduction of hip	

Medial Rotators of Hip

These muscles are the chief medial rotators of the hip joint (Table 1.5):
- Tensor fasciae latae
- Gluteus medius
- Gluteus minimus

Table 1.5: Medial rotators of hip joint					
Name	**Proximal attachment**	**Distal attachment**	**Innervation**	**Action**	
Tensor fasciae latae	External lip of the iliac crest between anterior superior iliac spine and tubercle of crest	Anterior aspect of the iliotibial tract	Superior gluteal nerve (L4, L5, S1)	By pulling the iliotibial tract, it assists gluteus maximus in extension of knee	
Gluteus medius	Gluteal surface of ilium between middle and posterior gluteal lines	Greater trochanter	Superior gluteal nerve (L4, L5, S1)	Abduction of hip	

Contd.

Table 1.5: Medial rotators of hip joint *(Contd.)*

Name	Proximal attachment	Distal attachment	Innervation	Action	
Gluteus minimus	Gluteal surface of ilium between middle and inferior gluteal lines	Greater trochanter	Superior gluteal nerve (L4, L5, S1)	Abduction of hip	

Lateral Rotators of Hip (Table 1.6)

These muscles cause lateral rotation of the thigh at the hip joint:
- Obturator externus
- Obturator internus
- Piriformis
- Superior gemellus
- Inferior gemellus
- Quadratus femoris

Name	Proximal attachment	Distal attachment	Innervation	Action	
Obturator externus	Obturator membrane and obturator foramen	Medial surface of greater trochanter	Posterior division of obturator nerve	Lateral rotation of hip	
Obturator internus	Internal surface of lateral wall of pelvis	Medial surface of greater trochanter	Nerve to obturator internus	Lateral rotation and abduction of hip	
Piriformis	Sacrum	Medial surface of greater trochanter	Anterior rami of S1, S2	External rotation of hip	

Table 1.6: Lateral rotators of hip joint

Contd.

Table 1.6: Lateral rotators of hip joint (*Contd.*)

Name	Proximal attachment	Distal attachment	Innervation	Action	
Superior gemellus	Spine of ischium	Obturator internus tendon	Nerve to obturator internus	Lateral rotation of hip	
Inferior gemellus	Ischial tuberosity	Obturator internus tendon	Nerve to quadratus femoris	Lateral rotation of hip	
Quadratus femoris	Ischial tuberosity	Intertrochanteric crest	Nerve to quadratus femoris	Lateral rotation and adduction of hip	

TRABECULAR PATTERN OF THE HIP

The bony trabeculae are dense cancellous bone which is deposited in a linear fashion to play, mainly a supportive role. The formation and the localization of bony trabeculae depends upon the forces of stress applied to the bone as per Wolff's law.

Wolff's Law

Wolff's law, postulated by Julius Wolff (1836–1902), states that bone in a healthy person or animal will adapt to the loads under which it is placed, i.e. the internal architecture of the trabeculae undergoes adaptive changes according to stresses. If the load is more, the trabeculae become thick and strong and if the load is less, the trabeculae become weak and thin.

The stresses responsible for trabecular pattern are both static and dynamic—static due to gravity and dynamic due to muscle action.

The configuration of the trabeculae at the upper end of femur is an apt example of Wolff's law and demonstrates the various forces, tensile or compressive, acting on the proximal end of the femur.

A coronal section of the proximal end of femur demonstrates the following sets of trabeculae:

- Principal compressive/medial compressive trabeculae
- Primary tensile trabeculae
- Secondary compressive/lateral compressive trabeculae
- Secondary tensile trabeculae
- Greater trochanteric trabeculae

These trabeculae at the proximal end of the femur are arranged in a particular pattern (Fig. 1.10).

This trabecular pattern at the upper end of the femur can be appreciated very well in a plain radiograph of the hip joint. Making use of this trabecular pattern, Singh and Singh (Manmohan Singh; AR Nagrath; PS Maini) from Rohtak, India have described an index (Fig. 1.11) in 1970, to assess the presence or absence of osteoporosis. They

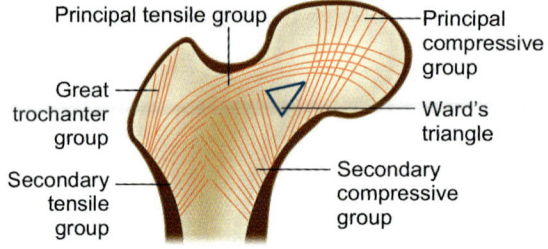

Fig. 1.10: Trabecular pattern of upper end of femur

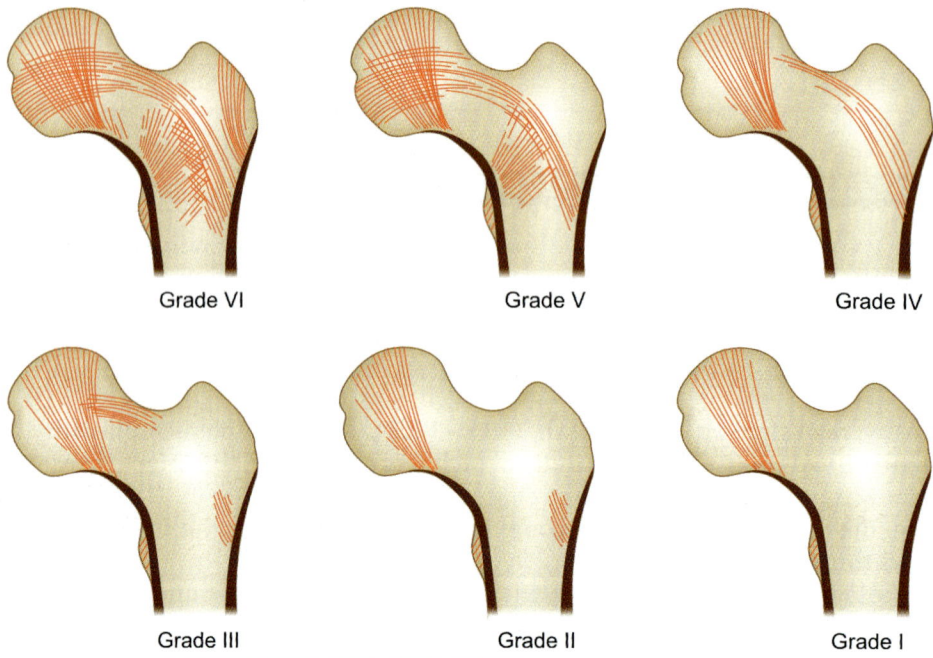

Grade VI

Grade V

Grade IV

Grade III

Grade II

Grade I

Fig. 1.11: Singh's index: Grade I–VI

have described 6 grades of bone density, as assessed by relative density of different trabeculae, seen in plain radiographs.

Grade VI is normal, and grade I is severe osteoporosis.

These grades are as follow.

Grade VI

- All normal trabecular groups are visible.
- Upper end of femur seems to be completely occupied by cancellous bone.

Grade V

- Principal tensile and principal compressive trabeculae are accentuated.
- Ward's triangle appears prominent.

Grade IV

- Principal tensile trabeculae are markedly reduced but can still be traced from lateral cortex to upper part of the femoral neck.

Grade III

- There is a break in the continuity of the principal tensile trabeculae opposite the greater trochanter.
- This grade indicates definite osteoporosis.

Grade II

- Only principal compressive trabeculae stand out prominently.
- Remaining trabeculae have been essentially absorbed.

Grade I

- Principal compressive trabeculae are markedly reduced in number and are no longer prominent over a period of years.
- The importance of this index has been overshadowed by more reliable and objective investigations like Dexa Scan. However, postgraduates of orthopaedics, particularly from India, must be aware of this index.

ANGULAR ORIENTATION OF UPPER END OF FEMUR AND ACETABULUM

Neck-Shaft Angle

The head and neck of femur are not in a straight line, but are at an angle. This angle can be measured accurately in an anteroposterior radiograph of the hip joint. Two lines are drawn—one line passing through mid axis of femur shaft, and another line passing along mid-axis of femoral neck and the centre of the head. The angle between these two lines is the neck-shaft angle (Fig. 1.12).

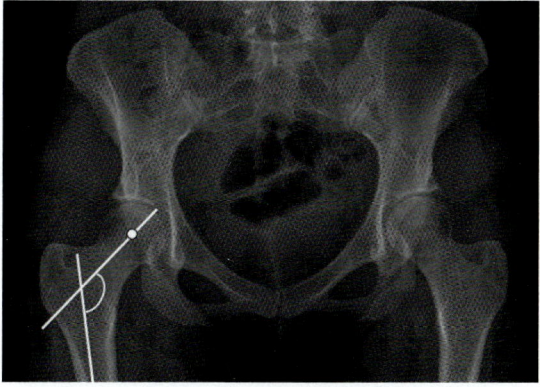

Fig. 1.12: Neck-shaft angle

Normal range of the neck-shaft angle is 120–135° in an adult.

In a newborn and an infant, this angle is more. In a newborn, the neck-shaft angle at the upper end of the femur is almost 150°. As the infant starts standing and walking, the neck-shaft angle starts reducing and by the age of 12 years, it comes to the final value of 120 to 135°.

In situations where neck-shaft angle is less than normal, i.e. below 120° it is called *coxa vara* (Fig. 1.13B). In instances where the neck-shaft angle is more than normal, i.e. more than 135°, is called *coxa valga* (Fig. 1.13C).

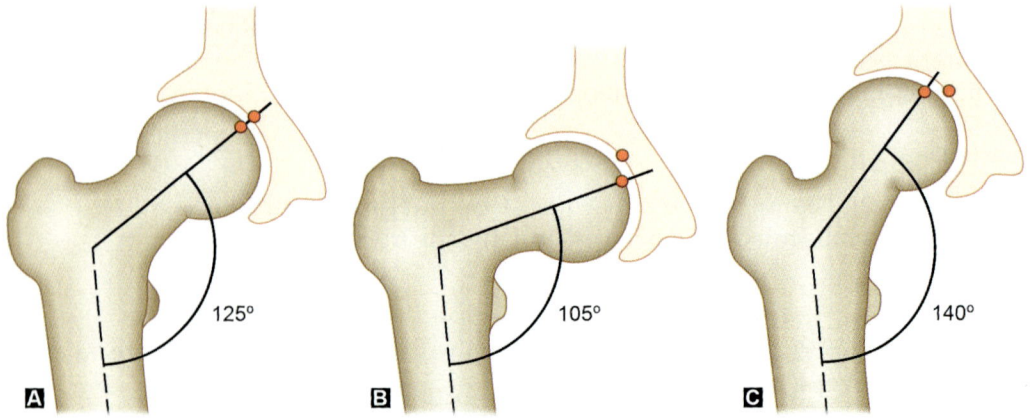

Fig. 1.13: Neck-shaft angle: **A.** Normal, **B.** Coxa vara, and **C.** Coxa valga

In either situation of coxa vara or coxa valga, the abductor mechanism of hip is disturbed and the patient's gait becomes abnormal, i.e. Trendelenburg gait.

Femoral Neck Anteversion

There is a unique anatomical configuration, which occurs at the proximal end of femur. The coronal plane of the shaft and distal part of femur, and the coronal plane of the head and neck of the femur are not coplanar—the coronal plane of the head and neck lies anterior to the coronal plane of shaft and distal femur, resulting in anteversion (Fig. 1.14).

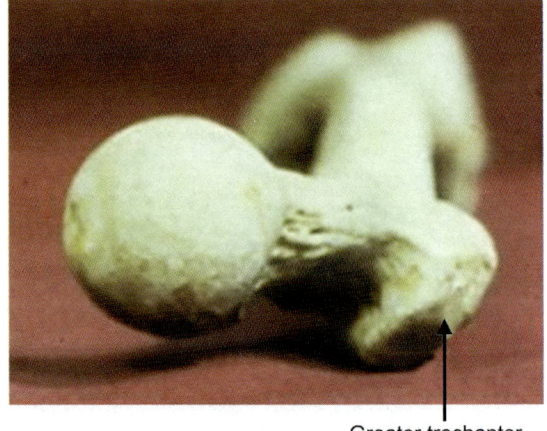

Greater trochanter

Fig. 1.14: Anteversion of head and neck (anatomical specimen)

Femoral neck anteversion can be assessed as the angle between an imaginary transverse line that runs from medial side to lateral side through the knee joint, and an imaginary transverse line passing through the centre of the femoral head and neck in a set-up where the image of head and neck segment is superimposed on the image of distal femur (Fig. 1.15).

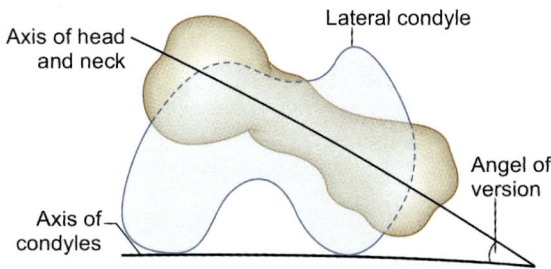

Fig. 1.15: Anteversion of neck (Image showing femoral neck superimposed on femoral condyles)

Normal range of anteversion is between 15° and 20°. In a situation where anteversion is increased, it manifests clinically as intowing. In the situation where anteversion is reduced, i.e. retroversion, it results in out-towing (Charlie Chaplin stance and gait) .

Acetabular Anteversion

The face of the acetabulum is not directed to a strict lateral position—it is directed anteriorly by about 15°. This results in an anatomical fact of anteversion of acetabulum (Fig. 1.16).

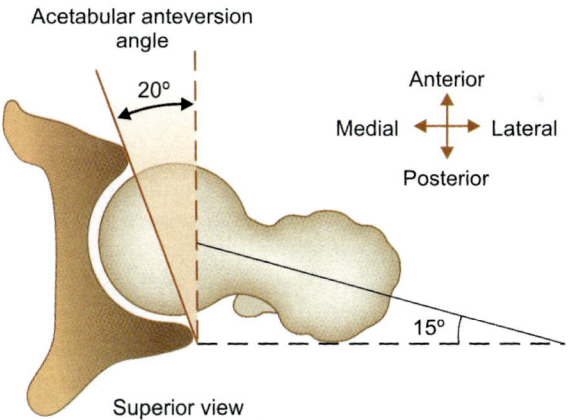

Fig. 1.16: Acetabular anteversion

The combined anteversion of neck of femur and acetabulum is responsible for the normal range of rotations (internal and external) of the hip.

BIOMECHANICAL FACTORS WORKING AROUND THE HIP

Out of the three types of lever mechanisms (Fig. 1.17), hip joint is a first order lever (Fig. 1.18) with forces on either side of fulcrum, i.e. body weight and abductor tension.

To maintain a stable hip joint, torque produced by the body weight is countered by abductor muscles pull.

Abductor force × lever arm A = Weight × lever arm B

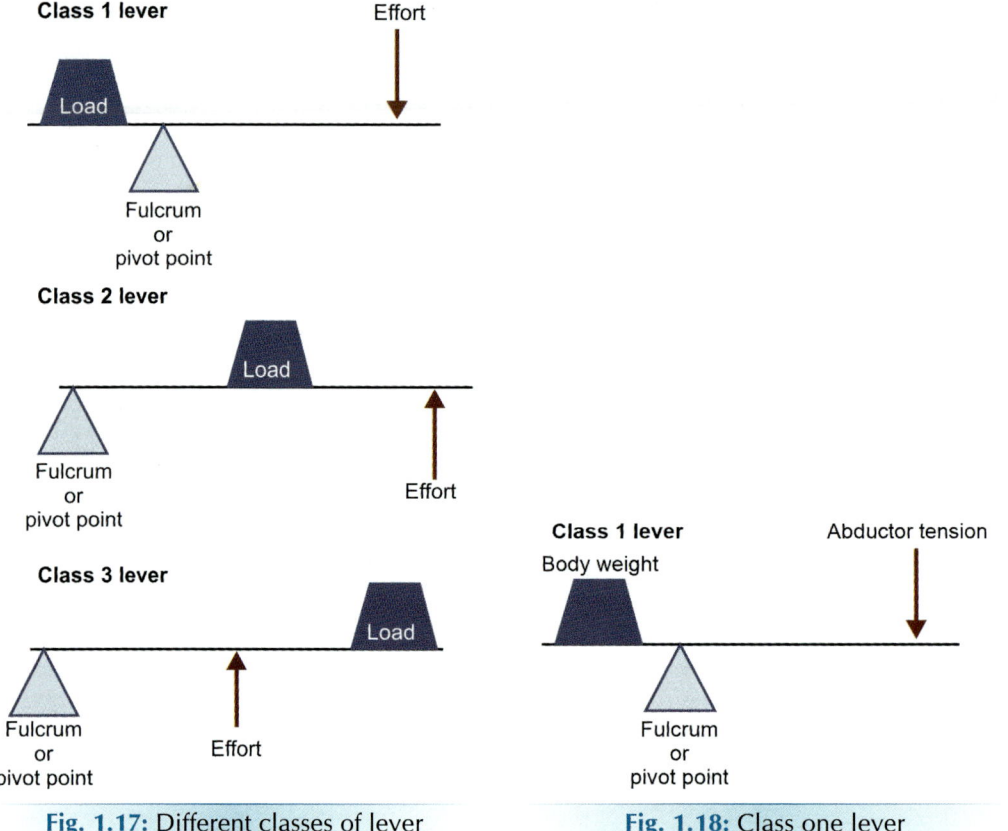

Fig. 1.17: Different classes of lever

Fig. 1.18: Class one lever

Joint Reaction Force

Joint reaction force (Fig. 1.19) is defined as force generated within a joint, in response to forces acting on the joint. In case of hip joint, the joint reaction force is generated in response to body weight and abductor muscle force.

Joint reaction force of the hip joint maintains the pelvis in a balanced position, without a tilt.

Joint reaction force can also be intepreted as the force resulting from the effort to maintain a balance between moment arms of the body weight and abductor tension.

The magnitude of joint reaction force (without going into detailed mathematical calculations) is enhanced significantly in different situations as depicted in Table 1.7.

Table 1.7: Joint reaction force in hip joint in different activities	
Stance/activity	*Magnitude of joint reaction force*
Straight leg raising	2W—twice the body weight
Single leg stance	3W—thrice the body weight
Walking	5W—5 times the body weight
Running	10W—10 times the body weight

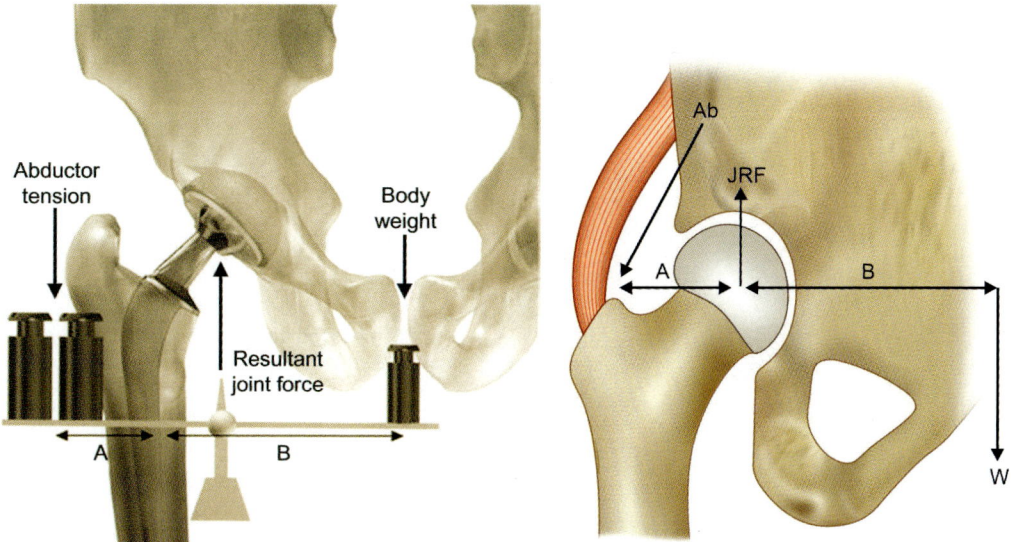

Fig. 1.19: Joint reaction force. Ab–Abductor force, A–Abductor moment arm, B–Moment arm of body weight, JRF–Joint reaction force, W–Body weight

Both Leg Stance

For the sake of simplicity and to make understanding easier, lower limbs constitute 2/6 of body weight and rest of the body (upper limbs and trunk) constitute 4/6.

The two hip joints support 4/6 or 2/3 of body weight (upper limbs and trunk) since both the hips are sharing equally 4/6 (2/3), each hip supports 1/3 of the body weight.

However, situation changes in the case of single leg stance as in walking and running.

Single Leg Stance

In a single leg stance (Fig. 1.20), the weight bearing hip would have to support weight of the trunk and upper limbs as well as weight of other lower limb. So the weight at the stance hip is equal to 4/6 +1/6 = 5/6. Effective centre of gravity shifts to the non-supportive leg and produces downward force to tilt pelvis.

Abductors on the stance phase side would have to produce a force to counteract 5/6 of the body weight which is trying to tilt the pelvis on the unsupported side.

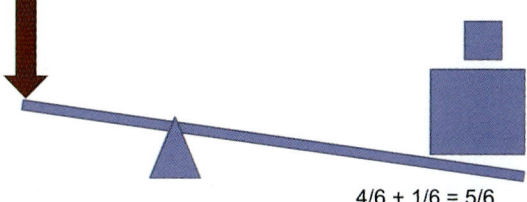

4/6 + 1/6 = 5/6

Fig. 1.20: Single leg stance: Abductors balance 5/6 of body weight

BLOOD SUPPLY OF FEMORAL HEAD

There has been some confusion in the mind of students in understanding the blood supply of the head of the femur, due to the varying nomenclature used by different authors describing the same artery (Fig. 1.21).

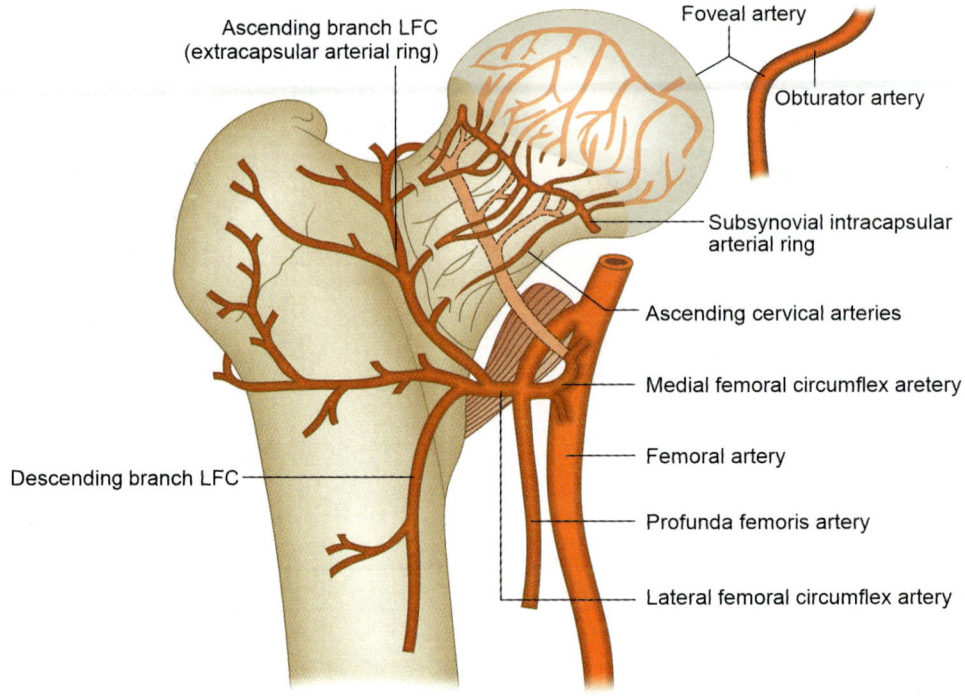

Fig. 1.21: Blood supply of femoral head

1. Gautier et al. and Kalhor et al. used the term retinacular arteries to describe the vessels passing in vicinity of retinacular fibres of capsule.
2. Treuta describes the same vessels as epiphyseal or metaphyseal depending upon which portion of bone they supplied, i.e. metaphysis or epiphysis during the growth period.
3. Crock and Chung described an extracapsular ring at the base of neck and an intracapsular ring at the base of head. The extracapsular ring giving the ascending cervical branches going along the neck of femur , which were called retinacular/ metaphyseal by other authors.

   However, some facts are without controversies which are as follows:
   - **The blood supply of femoral head is from:**
     1. Medial circumflex
     2. Lateral circumflex
     3. Inferior gluteal
     4. Superior gluteal and 1st perforating branch of profunda femoris.
        ✦ Medial circumflex supplies about 80% of the total blood supply.
        ✦ There is a ring which is extracapsular and is at the base of the neck of the femur. It is contributed to mainly by medial circumflex.
        ✦ Branches from this ring proceed from the neck surfaces and they have been variously called ascending cervical/metaphyseal/epihyseal/ retinacular.
        ✦ Lateral group of vessels which arise from the extra-articular ring are the most important and enter at the posterosuperior surface of neck.

+ The medial epiphyseal or the artery of ligamentum teres is a branch of obturator artery and is important in later stages of life.
+ Branches arising from the ring at the base probably lead to another intra-articular ring in the proximal part of neck of femur.

- **The blood supply of head of femur varies in different age groups**
  1. *At the time of birth*, all the vessels entering metaphysis and epiphysis anastomose freely, as the growth plate is absent. Artery of ligamentum teres is absent at birth.
  2. *4–7 years of age:* Growth plate has devloped. Artery of ligamentum teres has not devloped. Epiphyseal and metaphyseal arteries don't mix. Only supply of head of the femur (epiphysis) is from epiphyseal vessels. This is the most susceptible period for the epiphysis to develop avascular necrosis.
  3. *Adolscent:* Growth plate persists so that the anastomoses between metaphysis and epiphysis are poor. However, artery of ligamentum teres has developed, so head of the femur has dual blood supply.
  4. *Adult:* Growth plate disappears. All vessels anastomose. Main supply remains lateral group of branches arriving from the extracapsular ring.

2

Gait and Gait Analysis

✦ Normal gait (gait cycle)

✦ Phases of gait cycle

✦ Muscles involved in different phases of gait

✦ Joint position in different phases

✦ Common abnormal gaits

The manner of patient's walking, i.e. gait, can give important information about the underlying pathology of the diseased hip joint. Following prerequisites should be completed to make an adequate observation of a patient's gait.

1. Patient should be appropriately undressed with minimum essential clothes. In a male, he should be wearing only a T bandage or similar clothing to cover the perineal area. In a female, the breast area and the perineum should be adequately covered and a female attendant must be at hand.

2. Gait should be observed in an adequately lit corridor or area.

3. The clinician must observe the patient while:
   a. Patient is walking away from him for about 15–20 steps.
   b. Patient coming towards the clinician for about 15–20 steps.

Before understanding the deviations in the gait pattern in a case of hip disease, it will be appropriate first to know the features of normal gait.

NORMAL GAIT (GAIT CYCLE)

Definition

Normal gait cycle is a series of rhythmical, alternating movements of the trunk and limbs, which result in the forward progression of centre of gravity and the body. Nature has devised a very efficient-least energy consuming movements of the centre of gravity during normal gait. The progression of the centre of gravity is along a low amplitude sinusoidal pathway in the forward direction. Beside the forward progression movement, there is side-to-side movement also. This side-to-side movement is also along a sinusoidal path. The side-to-side movements of centre of gravity, which are inevitable during the normal gait, are also kept to a minimum (Fig. 2.1).

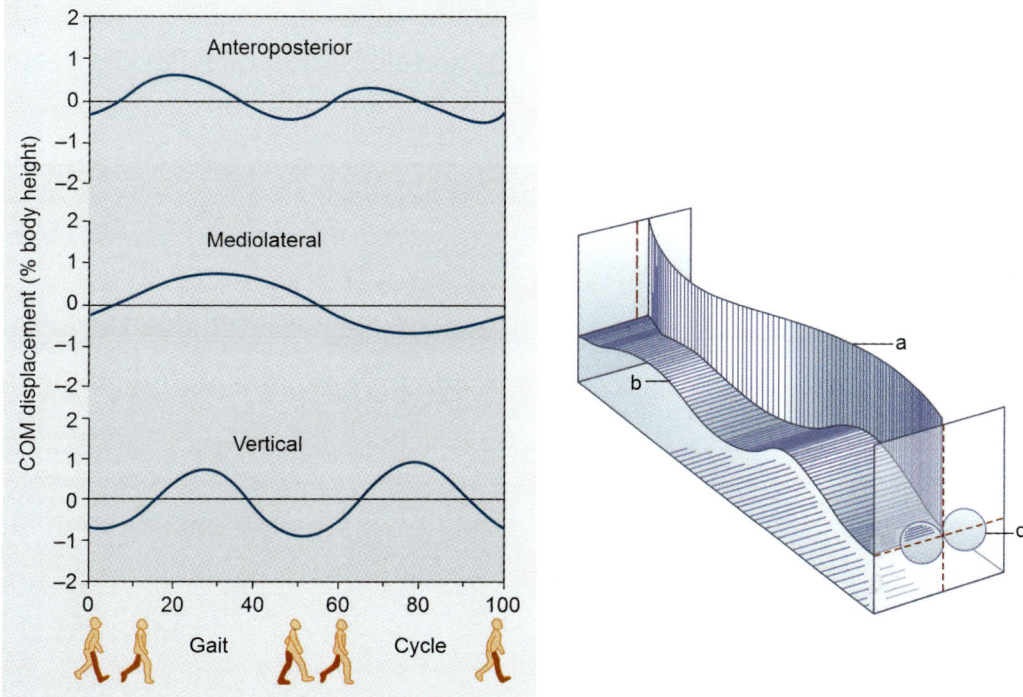

Fig. 2.1: Progression of centre of gravity: Sinusoidal curve in forward and side-to-side movements

PHASES OF GAIT CYCLE

Gait has been divided into two major phases:
1. Stance phase
2. Swing phase

Limb is supposed to be in stance phase when a part of the foot is in contact with the ground while in swing phase the foot is off the ground. The stance phase is 60% and swing phase accounts to 40% of gait cycle. The stance phase and swing phase have been further subdivided into different phases as shown in Table 2.1.

Table 2.1: Subdivisions of phases	
Stance phase	**Swing phase**
✖ Foot is on the ground	✖ When foot is off the ground, in air
✖ 60% of normal cycle is spent in stance phase (25% in double stance, i.e. both feet on the ground) 1. Heel strike 2. Foot flat: 7% 3. Mid-stance: 7–30% 4. Heel off: 30–40% 5. Toe off: 40–60%	✖ 40% of normal cycle 1. Acceleration: 60–75% 2. Mid-swing: 75–85% 3. Late swing: 85–100%

MUSCLES INVOLVED IN DIFFERENT PHASES OF GAIT

Different groups of muscles of joints of the lower limb act during different phases of the gait. Table 2.2 gives the summary of the activity of different muscles during different phases of the gait cycle.

Table 2.2: Muscles involved in different phases				
Phase	*Hip*	*Knee*	*Ankle*	
Heel strike	Flexion by rectus femoris	Extension by quadriceps	Controlled plantar flexion by eccentric contraction of tibialis anterior	
Foot flat	Extension by adductor magnus and gluteus maximus	Flexion by hamstrings	Controlled plantar flexion by eccentric contraction of tibialis anterior	
Mid-stance	Flexion by gluteus medius	Begins to extend by quadriceps	Supinated and dorsiflexed by triceps surae	

Contd.

Table 2.2: Muscles involved in different phases (*Contd.*)				
Phase	**Hip**	**Knee**	**Ankle**	
Push-off	Extension of hip by hamstrings	Knee in flexion by quadriceps	Plantar flexion by gastrocnemius and soleus	
Acceleration	Flexion by rectus femoris	Flexion by hamstrings	Dorsiflexion by tibialis anterior	
Mid-swing	Hip flexion by contraction of abductors	Knee flexion by sartorius	Dorsiflexion by tibialis anterior	
Deceleration	Hip flexion by abductors and hamstrings	Knee extension by quadriceps	Ankle in neutral position	

Different joints of the lower limb, i.e. hip, knee and ankle and foot, move in a definite pattern as the gait progresses. These three joints go through a well-defined change in their position during a normal gait cycle. The relative position of the different joints during the different phases of gait cycle is described below.

1. **Heel strike (initial contact):** This sub-phase begins at the moment, the foot touches the ground. It is also the first stage of double support.
   - There is 30° flexion of the hip (rectus femoris) and knee is in full extension (quadriceps).
   - Ankle moves from a neutral (supinated 5°) position into plantar flexion. (eccentric contraction of tibialis anterior).
2. **Foot flat (loading response phase)**
   - Body absorbs the impact of the foot.
   - Hip moves slowly towards extension (adductor magnus and gluteus maximus).
   - Knee flexes to 15–20° of flexion (hamstrings).
   - Ankle plantar flexion increases to 10–15°. (Eccentric elongation of dorsifexors, i.e. tibialis anterior)
3. **Mid-stance**
   - Body is supported by one leg.
   - Body begins to move from force absorption at impact to force propulsion forward.
   - Hip moves from 10° flexion to extension (gluteus medius).
   - Knee reaches maximal flexion (hamstrings) and then begins to extend (quadriceps).
   - Ankle becomes supinated and dorsiflexed (some contraction of triceps surae).
4. **Push-off**
   a. *Heel-off*
      - Begins when the heel leaves the floor.
      - Body weight is distributed over the metatarsal heads.
      - 10–13° of hip hyperextension which then moves towards flexion.
      - Knee becomes flexed (0–5°)
      - Ankle supinates and plantar flexes.
   b. *Toe-off*
      - The toes leave the ground.
      - Hip becomes less extended.
      - Knee is flexed 35–40°
      - Plantar flexion of ankle increases to 20°.
5. **Early swing (acceleration phase)**
   - Hip flexes to 20° with lateral rotation (contraction of rectus femoris muscle).
   - Knee flexes to 40–60°.
   - The ankle goes from 20° of plantar flexion to dorsiflexion by tibialis anterior.
6. **Mid-swing**
   - Hip flexes to 30° (contraction of hip abductors).
   - Ankle becomes dorsiflexed (tibialis anterior).
   - Knee flexes 60° (contraction of sartorius).

7. **Late swing (deceleration phase)**
   - Hip flexion by abductors and hamstrings.
   - Knee extension by quadriceps.
   - Ankle in neutral position.

JOINT POSITION IN DIFFERENT PHASES

Table 2.3 gives a summary of the joint position of the lower limb joints in a tabulated form.

Table 2.3: Joint position of lower limb				
Stance phase	**Hip**	**Knee**	**Ankle**	
Heel strike	30° flexion	Full extension and at the end knee flexion (5°) begins	Moves from a neutral (supinated 5°) position into plantar flexion	
Foot flat	Moves slowly into extension	Flexes to 15–20° of flexion	Plantar flexion increases to 10–15°	
Mid-stance	10° of flexion to extension	Reaches maximal flexion and then begins to extend	Supinated and dorsiflexed (5°)	

Contd.

Table 2.3: Joint position of lower limb (*Contd.*)

Stance phase	Hip	Knee	Ankle	
Push off				
a. Heel-off	10–13° of hip hyperextension, which then goes into flexion	Flexed (0–5°)	Supinates and plantar flexes	
b. Toe-off	Extended	Flexed 35–40°	Plantar flexion increases to 20°	
Acceleration	Hip extends to 20° and then flexes with lateral rotation	Flexes to 40–60°	20° of plantar flexion to dorsiflexion, to end in a neutral position	
Mid-swing	Flexes to 30°	flexes 60° but then extends approximately 30°	Dorsiflexed	

Contd.

Table 2.3: Joint position of lower limb (Contd.)				
Stance phase	**Hip**	**Knee**	**Ankle**	
Decelaration	Flexion of 25–30°	Locked extension	Neutral position	

COMMON ABNORMAL GAITS

Common abnormal gaits associated with hip diseases are:

1. Trendelenburg gait
2. Waddling gait
3. Antalgic gait
4. Short limb gait
5. Stiff hip gait

Other abnormal gaits like hand on thigh gait, hip hiking gait, wide-based gait, narrow-based gait, posterior trunk bending gait, etc. are mostly because of disease elsewhere.

Three major gaits are described below.

Trendelenburg Gait (Fig. 2.2)

Trendelenburg gait is consequent to disturbed abductor mechanism of the hip joint and can be found in a variety of hip pathologies. To understand this, one must know the abductor mechanism of hip joint, which constitutes of:

1. **Fulcrum:** Head of femur and acetabular socket
2. **Lever arm:** Neck of femur and trochanteric region
3. **Power:** Primarily gluteus medius aided by tensor fasciae latae

The abductor mechanism is responsible for preventing the fall of the unsupported hemipelvis due to gravity, on the side which is non-weight-bearing, i.e. the lower limb on that side is in swing phase. To understand it more clearly, one must appreciate the sequence of events in one leg stance.

In one-legged stance, either during normal walking or if the patient is specifically asked to stand on one leg, the hemipelvis on the unsupported limb tends to go down because of gravity. In a normal person, this tendency of unsupported pelvis to go down is counteracted by abductors of the contralateral hip joint or the limb which is in stance phase, i.e. weight-bearing limb. These contralateral abductors on the stance phase limb side contract at their pelvic attachment (not the trochanteric attachment or insertion). This contraction helps to prevent sagging of the hemipelvis on the unsupported side. One must understand that if patient is standing on the right foot, i.e. right lower limb is in stance phase and the left lower limb is in the air or swing phase, the tendency of the left-sided hemipelvis to sag down is counteracted by the intact right-sided abductors.

If the patient has a disease of the right hip—when right lower limb is in stance phase and left side is in swing phase, the left side will sag down. The patient tries

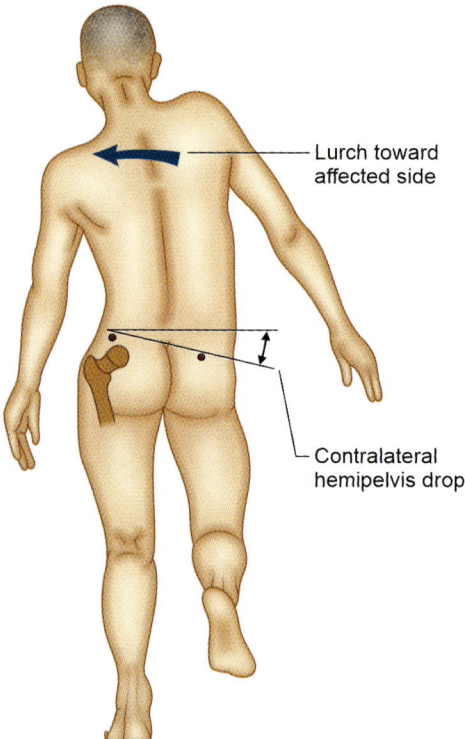

Lurch toward
affected side

Contralateral
hemipelvis drop

Fig. 2.2: Trendelenburg gait

to counteract this by bending or lurching the trunk towards the right side to partly prevent sagging of the left hemipelvis. This results in positive Trendelenburg sign and consequently Trendelenburg gait.

Any disruption of the abductor mechanism in any of its three parts will result in Tredelenburg gait. Therefore, the causes of Trendelenburg gait are:

1. **Defective fulcrum:** Dislocation of hip, DDH, Perthes disease, osteonecrosis of femoral head
2. **Defective lever system:** Neck of femur fractures, trochanteric avulsion, coxa vara
3. **Diseased abductors:** Poliomyelitis, muscular dystrophies, L5 radiculopathy, cerebral palsy.

Waddling Gait

If the abductor mechanism of both hip joints is affected, then patient lurches alternatively on the side which is in stance phase. This leads to waddling gait or 'duck walk gait'. Common conditions leading to this gait are bilateral AVN, bilateral DDH and myopathy paralysis of abductors of both hips. However, it has also been observed in pregnancy and patients of osteomalacia.

Antalgic Gait

Antalgic gait (Fig. 2.3) is seen when the patient attempts to avoid putting weight on one leg due to pain anywhere from hip to foot, i.e. besides hip pathology, it can be seen in diseases of other parts of lower limb also.

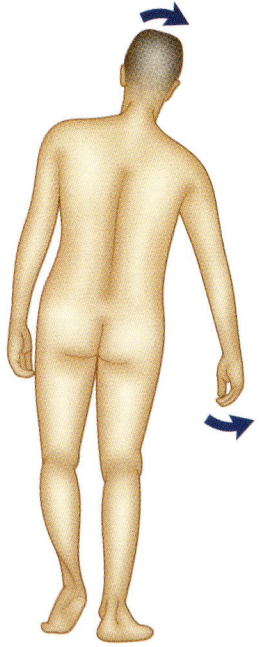

Fig. 2.3: Antalgic gait

The primary sign of antalgic gait is the reduced amount of time spent in stance phase. This is because the patient experiences pain in stance phase, and tries to spend minimum time in a painful situation. Besides reduced stance phase, one can also observe decreased stride length in a case of antalgic gait.

Some other additional features can also be seen in antalgic gait, like grimace on the face of patient, exaggerated movements of upper extremities when the painful element is severe.

Short Limb Gait (Fig. 2.4)

If one limb is short because of some disease, as the patient walks, the affected side of the body dips down in order to make it possible to bring the foot to the ground. In other words, the head of the patient, trunk and the pelvis drops on the affected side in the stance phase. So the characteristics of a short limb gait are up and down movements of one-half of the body.

- Initially, if the shortening is less than 1.5 cm, typical short limb gait may not be apparent as it is compensated by pelvic tilt and there is no real fall of trunk and head while walking.

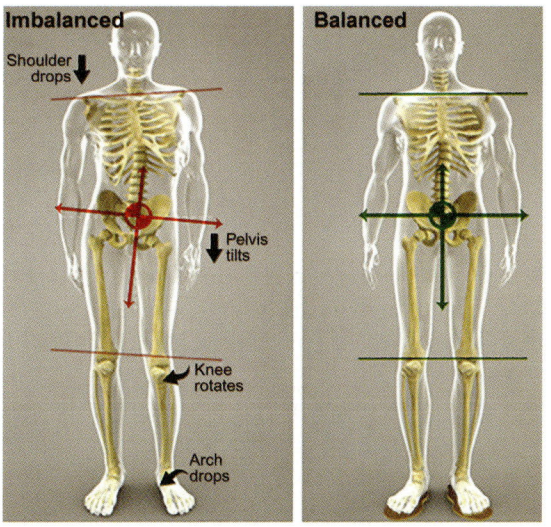

Fig. 2.4: Short limb gait

- If shortening is 1.5–4 cm, it is compensated by hyperextension at the knee and equinus at the ankle.
- The typical short limb gait is seen when the shortening is more than 4 cm.

Stiff Hip Gait (Fig. 2.5)

Another type of pathological gait which may be seen in cases of advanced hip pathology is stiff hip gait or ankylosed hip gait (Fig. 2.5). Normally, there is forward rotation of the pelvis in the swing phase. This rotation of the pelvis on the swing phase side occurs around the fulcrum of the lower limb which is in stance phase. If the hip on the stance phase side is stiff, i.e. movements are absent or negligible, the swinging, rotational, forward movement of the pelvis of the extremity in swing phase are defective and lack rhythm. The forward rotation of the pelvis, which is essential for forward progression of the body, occurs around the fulcrum of stable knee, foot and ankle in place of the hip.

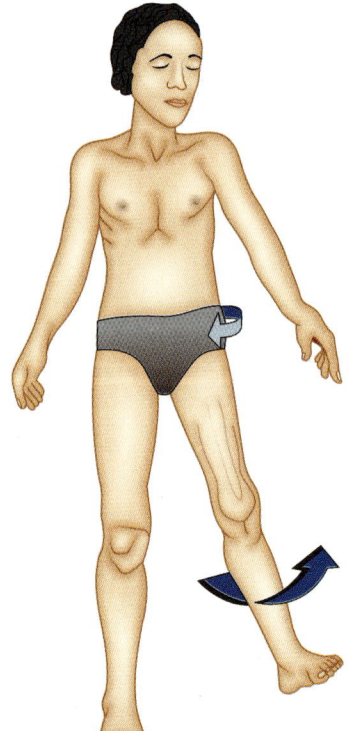

Fig. 2.5: Ankylosed hip gait

Further when the hip is ankylosed it is not possible to flex the hip joint during gait cycle to clear the ground during swing phase. Therefore, the person with stiff hip lifts the pelvis on that side and swings the leg with the pelvis in circumduction and moves it forward.

This gait is also described as circumduction or hip hiking gait.

CHAPTER

3

Introduction to
Hip Examination

✦ History ✦ Examination

Hip joint examination is important for any postgraduate student because he/she is likely to get a case of hip joint disease as a long case in practical examination. At the same time, hip joint examination is no less important for a qualified orthopaedic surgeon, since patient of hip joint disease form a major part of orthopaedic practice. It is important for residents as well as consultants in orthopaedics to learn, understand and master the hip joint examination.

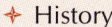 **HISTORY**

The importance of an adequate history preceding the hip joint examination cannot be overemphasized. From an accurate history, strong clues are available for final diagnosis. Important points to be elaborated in history would be:

1. **Pain**
   a. *Location:* Hip pain is mostly anterior, while pain of spine origin is posterior in gluteal area.
   b. *Type of pain:* Pain can be acute like in transient synovitis of hip joint, septic arthritis or trauma, or chronic, as in cases of tuberculosis.
   c. *Severity of pain:* It could be mild like in Perthes disease or severe as in cases of inflammatory arthritis. History of night pains is important. It classically occurs in tuberculosis when following suppression of muscle spasm during sleep, the articular cartilages touch and cause sudden pain which wakes up the patient.
   d. *Aggravating factors* like weight bearing, as in osteoarthritis or initial stages of tuberculosis, secondary arthritis, etc.
2. **Limp:** The clinician should enquire, if the patient is able to walk normally or not. Does he require a walking aid, like cane or crutch? If so, he should also enquire on which side the patient is using the walking aid, ipsilateral or contralateral. If the patient is able to walk without support, does he have a limp or not? If a patient of hip disease is ambulatory, a limp or pathological gait is almost always present.
3. **Limb length discrepancy:** Majority of patients of chronic hip joint disease would complain of shortening because of articular cartilage loss or bone destruction. In a very small percentage, patient may complain of lengthening as in case of initial stage of hip joint tuberculosis.

4. **Fever:** Presence of fever, particularly if moderate or high, indicates presence of an infective process. Mild fever can be seen in RA or other chronic non-infective inflammatory pathologies. One can also enquire about whether fever comes concomitantly with pain or swelling, whether it is continuous or intermittent. Continuous low-grade fever with evening rise of temperature is a feature of tuberculosis.

5. **Ability to squat and sit cross-legged:** This is of particular importance for patients from the Asian subcontinent, because of prevalent professional and religious practices.

6. **Medication/treatment taken:** One should specifically ask for intake of steroids, antitubercular treatment in the past and any operation done in past or a distant history of trauma.

7. **Involvement of spine and other joint:** Involvement of spine and other joint indicates a systemic/polyarticular disease, the commonest being ankylosing spondylitis.

By any standards, the above list is not complete/comprehensive, since the author is focused mainly on examination of the hip joint.

EXAMINATION

The examination should be undertaken in a sufficiently lit room and after undressing the patient appropriately. Availability of a couch with a firm mattress to examine the hip joint is basic requirement. A male patient can be examined after reassuring the patient and dressing him in a loin cloth or a T-bandage only. Examination of a female patient should be performed in presence of a female attendant/staff nurse; and by taking care to appropriately cover the perineum and breasts. Needless to say, the patient must be taken into confidence. Availability of a goniometer, percussion hammer, measuring tape, marker pen are some basic requirements for hip examination. A plumb line may also be sometimes required.

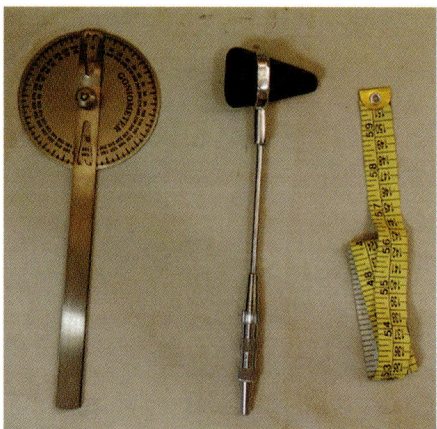

Fig. 3.1: Instruments required in examination

Examination of hip joint should proceed in a definite sequence, which is as follows:

1. Inspection
2. Palpation
3. Movements
4. Measurements
5. Special tests

4

Inspection

Inspection should proceed in the following sequence:
1. Gait
2. Inspection while standing
3. Inspection from back
4. Inspection from side
5. Inspection in supine position
    a. Attitude
    b. Skin condition
    c. Muscular wasting or atrophy
    d. swelling
    e. Scar marks
    f. Sinus
    g. Ulcers
    h. Pulsations
    i. Contractures
    j. Fixed bony points.

GAIT

If the patient is able to walk and allowed to walk, the examining doctor should make a note whether the patient is walking normally or with some assistance. The abnormal gait patterns commonly seen are Trendelenburg, short limb, and antalgic gait, which have been previously described in Chapter 2.

After the gait examination, the patient is inspected in the standing and lying down position. In the standing position, the patient is observed (inspected) from the front, side and the back. When observing from side, one must note lumbar lordosis.

INSPECTION WHILE STANDING

The patient is examined from front, side and back.

While inspecting from the front (Fig. 4.1), following things should be noted:
    a. Head is central or not
    b. Shoulders at the same level or not
    c. Position of ASIS
    d. Symmetry of lateral margins of body

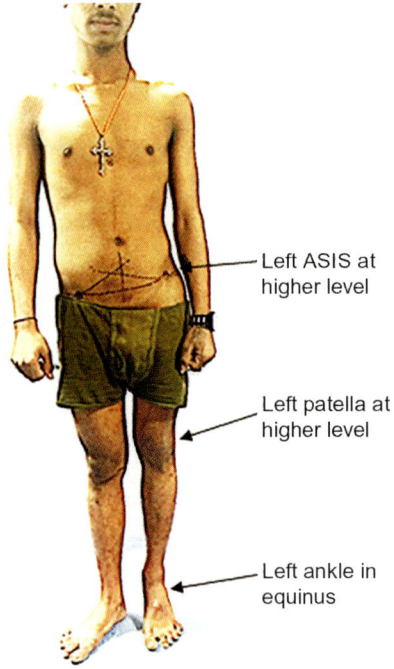

Fig. 4.1: Inspection from front

Left ASIS at higher level

Left patella at higher level

Left ankle in equinus

e. Level of patella, medial malleoli and feet
f. Any obvious scar, ulcer, redness, etc.

INSPECTION FROM BACK (Fig. 4.2)

Following observations are made.

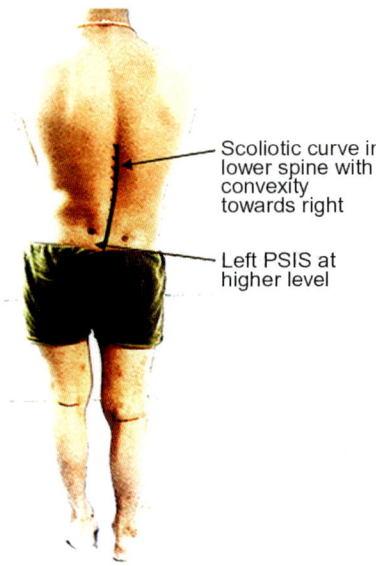

Scoliotic curve in lower spine with convexity towards right

Left PSIS at higher level

Fig. 4.2: Inspection from behind

a. Head is central or not
b. Shoulders level or not
c. Spine is straight or not
d. Lateral margins of body
e. Level of dimples of Venus
f. Level of iliac crests
g. Wasting of gluteus mass and posterior thigh bulk

INSPECTION FROM SIDE (Fig. 4.3)

The significant observation which should be specifically made is whether the normal dorsal kyphosis and lumbar lordosis are maintained or not. Normally there is 20–40° of lumbar lordosis. Exaggerated lumbar lordosis is seen in hip diseases because of presence of fixed flexion deformity of the hip joint. There is forward pelvic tilt as a compensatory mechanism to counteract flexion deformity of hip joint. If the hip joint is fixed in flexion, limb will be in the air unless it is brought down by compensatory movements at the lower lumbar spine and resultant tilt of the pelvis and bringing the foot to the ground. These compensatory movements at lower lumbar spine manifest as exaggerated lumbar lordosis which can be made out easily.

A physiological increase in lumbar lordosis may be observed during pregnancy and in any other situation where there is protuberant abdomen, like obesity, ascites, weak abdominal muscles, etc.

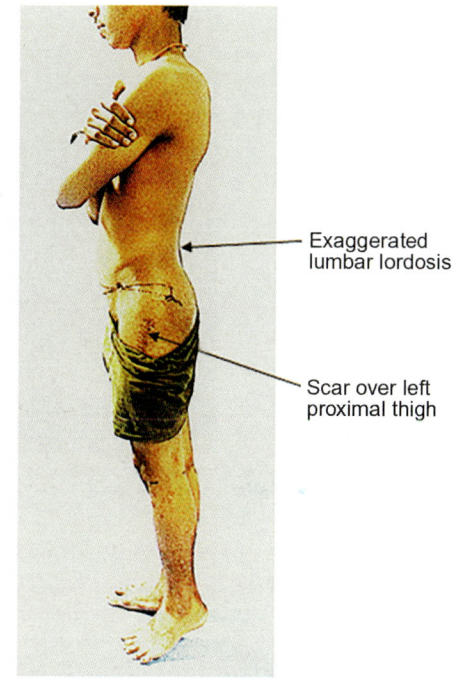

Exaggerated lumbar lordosis

Scar over left proximal thigh

Fig. 4.3: Inspection from side

INSPECTION IN LYING DOWN POSITION

Observe following things:
a. **Attitude of limb:** Attitude of the limb can vary in different stages of the same disease and also in different diseases of hip. The attitude may vary among rotation (internal/external)/abduction/adduction/flexion (hip lying in attitude of extension has not been described).

Different hip diseases may have a combination of all these attitudes. Common hip pathologies and attitude of limb in those pathologies are listed below (Fig. 4.4A):
- *Intertrochanteric fracture:* Marked external rotation of the foot is present, with the lateral border of foot touching the couch (Fig. 4.4A).
- *Neck of femur fracture:* The limb is in external rotation. However, compared to the marked external rotation attitude seen in intertrochanteric fractures, the

external rotation is less because of the intra-articular fracture and restraining effect of the capsule of the hip joint.

- *Synovial effusion of hip joint:* Flexion, abduction and external rotation altitude, which results in an appearance of lengthening of the lower limb, is seen in transient synovitis of hip and in cases of tuberculosis (Fig. 4.4A).
- *Arthritis of hip:* In a case of arthritis of the hip joint, which by definition is involvement of articular cartilage, there is an attitude of flexion, adduction and internal rotation (Fig. 4.4B). The arthritis may be because of various aetiologies, like tuberculosis, rheumatoid arthritis, post-traumatic arthritis, etc.

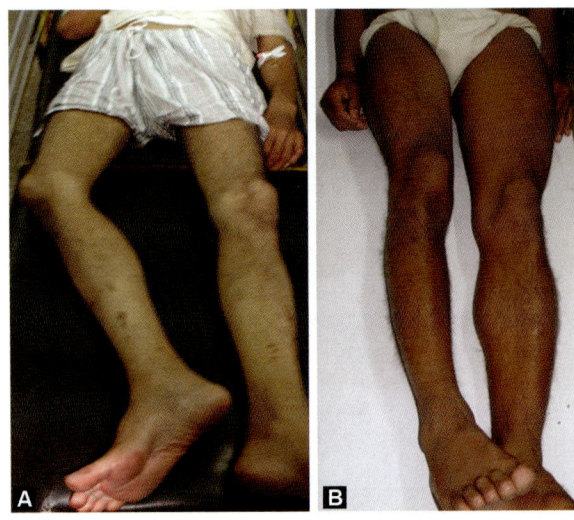

Fig. 4.4A and B: Attitude of limb: (A) Patella facing outward; (B) Patella facing inward

- *Posterior dislocation of hip:* Flexion, adduction and internal rotation with shortening.
- *Anterior dislocation of hip:* Flexion, abduction and external rotation with lengthening.

b. **Skin condition, like colour, stretching, etc.:** Inflamed skin indicates underlying infection. Since the hip joint is a deep-seated joint, the condition of the skin may not be affected in most of the cases. Skin may uncommonly be involved in a hip joint disease, either because of basic pathology which is affecting both the hip and skin like rheumatoid arthritis or in very late stages of disease when the pus/effusion has ruptured the capsule. In a patient of trauma or local abrasion, rarely a Morel-Lavallée lesion of subcutaneous haematoma may be seen in a fresh case of hip fracture.

c. **Muscular wasting/atrophy:** Wasting of quadriceps or gluteal region must be made a note of, it indicates a chronic disease. In India, tubercular hip arthritis is a common cause of gross wasting. Classically, wasting observed in cases of tuberculosis is described as disproportionate, i.e. wasting much more than expected from stage of disease.

d. **Swelling:** Swelling in vicinity of hip joint may be because of an enlarged lymph node in the inguinal area, pus formation (pyogenic or tubercular), post-traumatic haematoma and uncommonly dislocated bony head or a tumour arising from the neighbouring bone.

e. **Scar marks:** Make a note of a surgical scar mark or healing by secondary intention and exact anatomical position of the scar.

f. **Sinuses** in vicinity of hip joint occur mostly in cases of infective arthritis. The sinus may develop either primarily, or uncommonly after surgical intervention.

g. **Ulcers** are rarely seen in hip pathology.

h. **Pulsations:** More of academics interest; visual pulsations are rarely seen on inspection.

i. **Contracture around the hip joint** is mostly seen in post polio residual paralysis (fortunately rarely seen nowadays).

j. **Level of fixed bony points** (Fig. 4.5A and B)

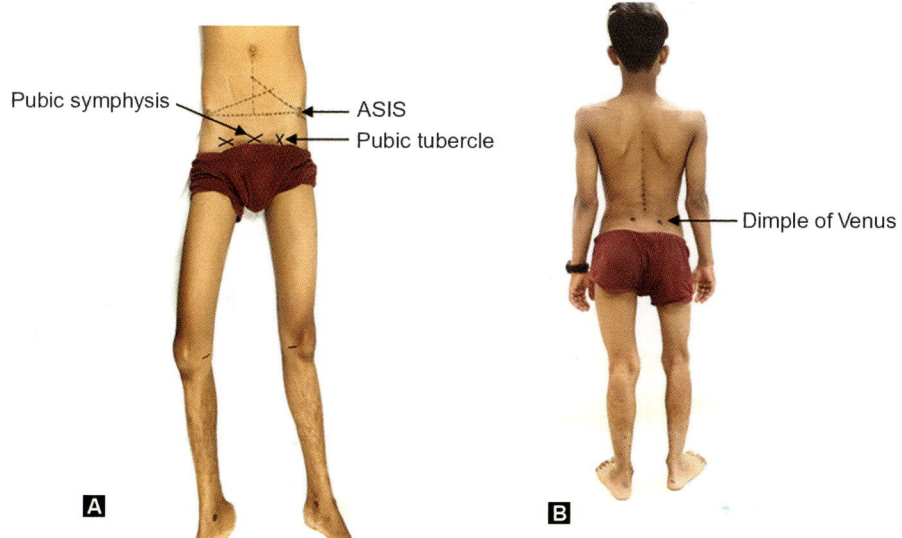

Fig. 4.5A and B: Bony points, on inspection: (A) From front; (B) From back

Bony points are ultimately assessed on palpation; however, few bony points can be commented in inspection—anterior superior iliac spine (front), trochanter (side), posterior superior iliac spine (dimple of Venus—back). One should make an observation of the level of above bony points as compared to the normal side.

5

Palpation

GENERAL PALPATION

At the start of palpation, two things are to be tested first before any other palpatory examination (as everywhere else in medicine).

1. **Local temperature should be assessed by dorsum of hand** (Fig. 5.1).
2. **Tenderness:** Any tenderness has to be elicited. The tenderness could be either superficial or deep.
   a. *Superficial tenderness:* Superficial tenderness may be felt in cases of abscess formation, inflammatory bursitis like trochanteric bursitis, avulsion of the muscles—most commonly adductor longus.

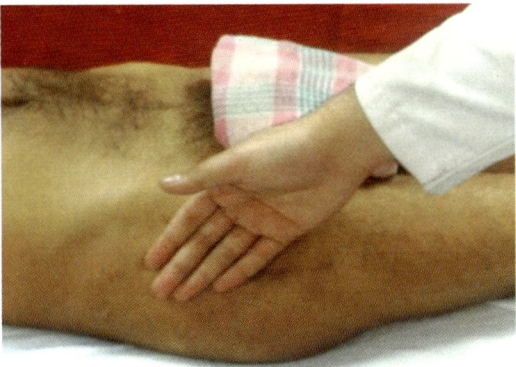

Fig. 5.1: Check for temperature using dorsum of hand

   b. *Deep tenderness:* It is elicited in the following manners:
      i. *Anterior hip joint tenderness:* To check for tenderness of hip joint, palpate just 1 cm below and lateral to the midpoint of inguinal ligament. This point will also be just lateral to femoral artery pulsations (Fig. 5.2).
      ii. *Trochanteric tenderness:* Tenderness will be present laterally over trochanter in cases of trochanteric fractures, osteomyelitis, neoplastic lesion, bursitis or other inflammatory conditions.

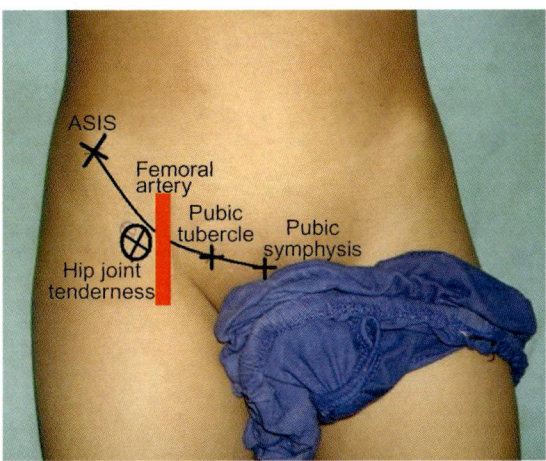

Fig. 5.2: Tenderness of hip joint

iii. *Bitrochanteric compression test:* In this manoeuvre, tenderness is elicited centrally in the hip joint, or in its vicinity by compressing both greater trochanters simultaneously. Tenderness elicited indicates central hip pathology, since the force is transmitted from trochanter to hip joint. It may be present in cases of acetabular fractures, and infections (Fig. 5.3).

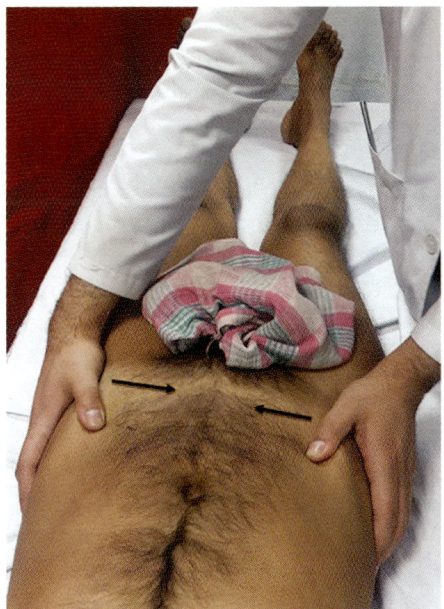

Fig. 5.3: Bitrochanteric compression test

It is important to mark certain bony points around the hip joint, which will be helpful in the examination:

• *Anterior superior iliac spine (ASIS):* It can be felt as the first bony prominence on moving the fingertips along the inguinal ligament in upward and lateral direction and marking the point (Fig. 5.4).

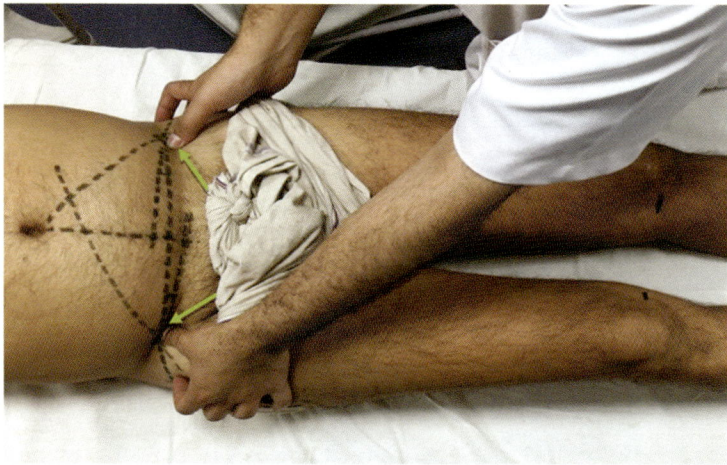

Fig. 5.4: Palpation of ASIS

- *Iliac crests:* If one keeps the thumb on the ASIS and let the fingers go along the bone from the ASIS in a posterior direction, one can appreciate and delineate the iliac crest. About 7.5 cm (3 inches) from the ASIS lies the iliac tubercle at the widest part of the crest.

  It will not be out of place to remind that the highest point of iliac crest lies between spinous process of L4–L5.
- *Pubic symphysis:* Pubic symphysis can be identified by moving fingertips downwards from umbilicus in the centre till bony point is felt.
- *Pubic tubercles:* These are situated about 2.5 cm on either side of pubic symphysis. Their position can also be confirmed by tracing the inguinal ligament medially.
- *Greater trochanter:* The tip of greater trochanter can be identified by palpating the shaft of the femur and moving the fingertips in proximal direction till a dip is appreciated where the bone ends (Figs 5.5 to 5.7). The Greater trochanter can also be appreciated by keeping the thumbs on the two anterior superior iliac spines and the fingers of the respective hands on either iliac crest and then moving the fingertips gradually downwards and

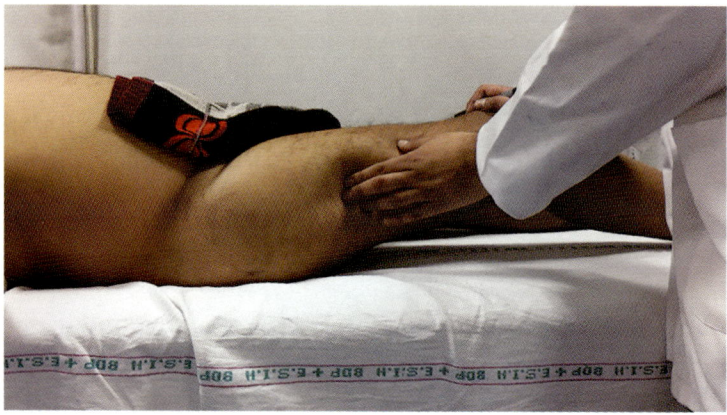

Fig. 5.5: Marking of greater trochanter—palpating shaft of femur

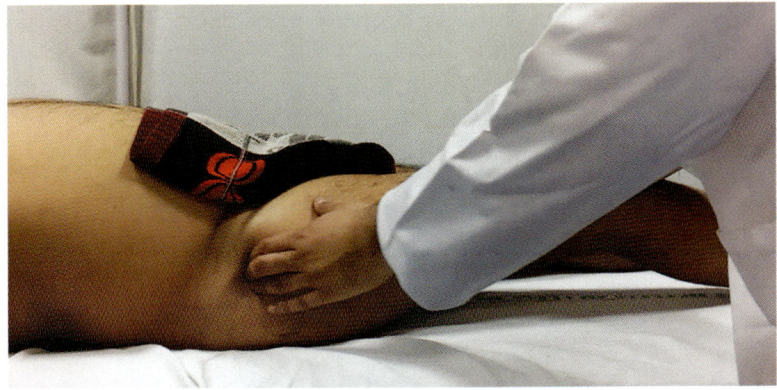

Fig. 5.6: Marking of greater trochanter—dip is felt proximal to tip of greater trochanter

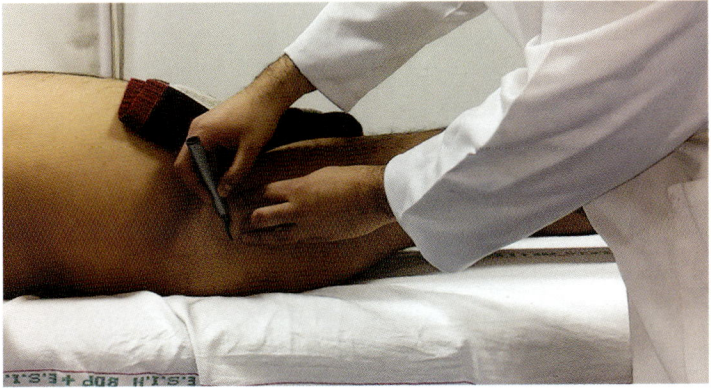

Fig. 5.7: Greater trochanter is marked where dip is felt

laterally to feel the trochanteric mass. One can appreciate that the posterior border of the greater trochanter is easily palpable while the lateral surface, anterior border and even the tip are covered by muscles and are not so palpable.

- *Posterior superior iliac spine (PSIS)* (Fig. 5.8)*:* It is represented by dimple of Venus on each side of vertebral column. The plane joining the two PSIS passes through S2 vertebra and middle of SI joint.

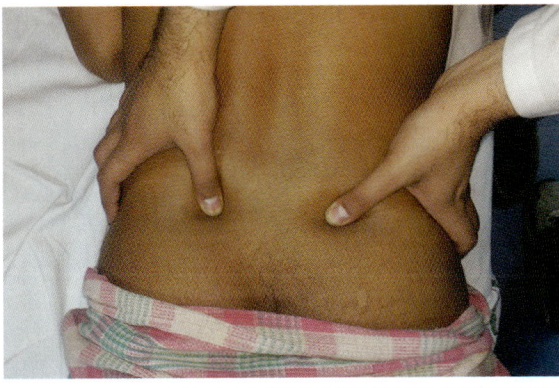

Fig. 5.8: PSIS—represented by dimple of Venus on each side

- *Ischial tuberosity:* It is felt as a bony protuberance at the site of gluteal fold. In neutral and extended position of the hip, it is not well palpable because of the overlying gluteus maximus mass. It can be better appreciated on flexing the hip. In the normal anatomical position, the level of ischial tuberosity corresponds to the lesser trochanter (Fig. 5.9).

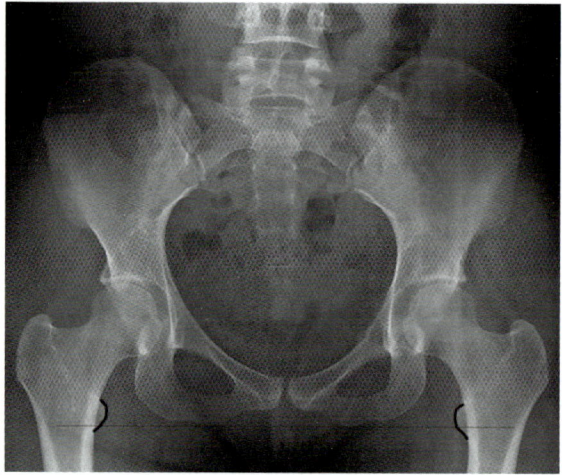

Fig. 5.9: Ischial tuberosity lies at the level of lesser trochanter

3. **Vascular sign of Narath:** Femoral artery pulsation is nicely palpable against the hard surface of underlying head of femur covered by tough fibrous capsule. It is best palpable by slightly flexing, abducting and external rotating the limb on the side being examined (Fig. 5.10).

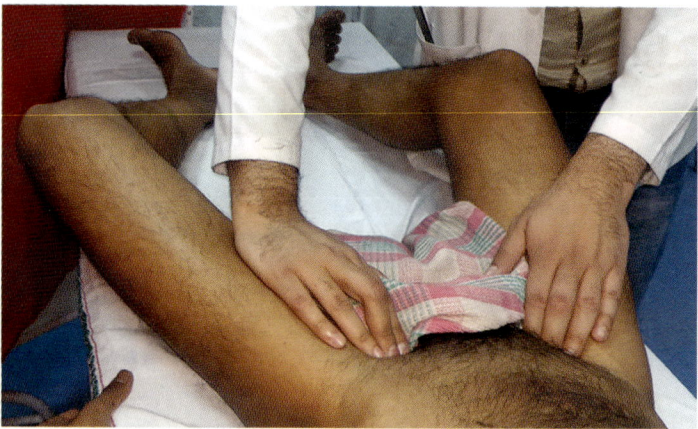

Fig. 5.10: Vascular sign of Narath

This test is performed by palpating the femoral pulsations on both sides simultaneously. The test is said to be positive, if the femoral pulsation is absent or felt less (reduced) on one side as compared to the other side. The test is positive in case of dislocation of hip joint, and gross destruction of the femoral head. One should understand that femoral pulse in most of the cases will not be totally absent in cases of hip dislocation. It will be palpable feebly against the tough fibrous capsule, beneath which the head of femur is absent.

4. **A swelling or a cold abscess** should be ruled out. Following sites should be inspected for any collection from hip joint or cold abscess:
   - Base of Scarpa's triangle
   - Gluteal region
   - Supratrochanteric region
   - Iliac fossa
   - Anteromedial aspect of mid-thigh (up to the knee in that direction)

5. **Digital Bryant's triangle:** As part of the palpation, one must assess relative proximal migration of the greater trochanter in a case of hip pathology. This can be done by creating a triangle with the help of thumb and two adjacent fingers in the following manner.

   The tip of thumb is kept at anterior superior iliac spine, tip of middle finger at tip of greater trochanter and tip of index finger at a point on the skin where a vertical drawn from anterior superior iliac spine towards the couch will intersect an imaginary line going proximally from the tip of the trochanter. Both the sides should be palpated simultaneously in this manoeuvre, to make the comparison easy. The distance between the tip of index and middle fingers, which is also the base of the triangle, is assessed visually. The base would be smaller on the affected side, indicating that tip of greater trochanter on that side has migrated proximally (Figs 5.11 and 5.12).

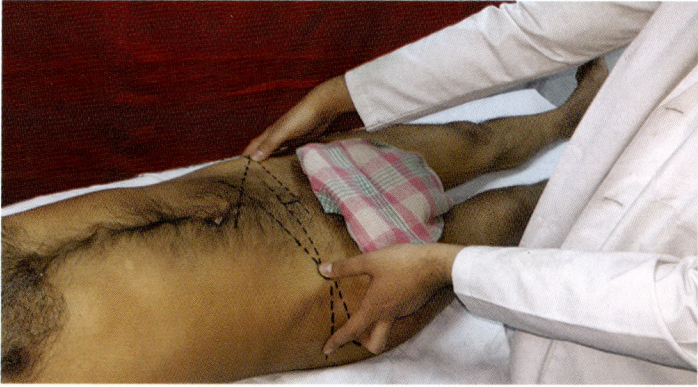

Fig. 5.11: Digital Bryant's triangle

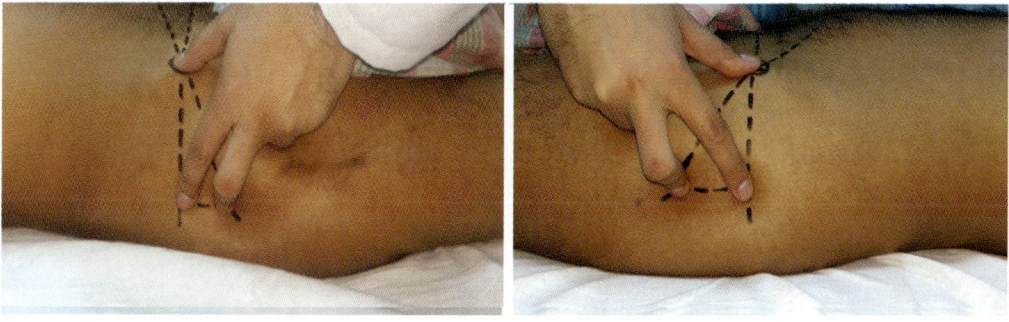

Fig. 5.12: Digital Bryant's triangle showing proximal migration of greater trochanter on right side

6. **Crepitus:** Try to feel for any crepitus, particularly near the trochanter. Crepitus may be felt in a fresh or old fractures.

FIXED DEFORMITIES OF HIP JOINT

In examination of the hip joint, palpation has got a special part/characteristic, which is regarding the assessment of different fixed deformities of the hip.

In a case of any fixed hip joint deformity, it is meant that the hip joint is fixed in that position because of the disease process. Hip joint can be fixed in flexion position, abduction/adduction and internal/external rotation. Movement of the hip joint in a direction opposite to that of the fixed deformity will be absent— for example, in a case of fixed flexion deformity of hip joint, the hip cannot be moved in the direction of extension from the point of fixed flexion deformity. Similarly in a case where the hip joint is fixed in external rotation, internal rotation would be absent beyond the fixed external rotation deformity. In a hip fixed in adduction, the hip joint cannot be moved in the direction of abduction beyond the fixed adduction deformity.

Assessment of Fixed Flexion Deformity

An exaggerated lumbar lordosis, observed during inspection should forewarn the examiner that there is likelihood of fixed flexion deformity. Before learning the method of measuring fixed flexion deformity, one must understand the pathogenesis of increased lumbar lordosis, seen in cases of fixed flexion deformity of hip joint.

Mechanism of Development of Exaggerated Lordosis in Fixed Flexion Deformity

When a hip joint is fixed in flexion, the limb and the foot is away from the ground in a position of flexion. For the purpose of ambulation and walking, the foot which would be in air (consequent to flexed position of hip) must be brought down to the ground. Since the movement of extension is not possible in the fixed and flexed hip, this is achieved by the patient by compensatory movements at the lower lumbar spine. There occurs hyperextension of the lower lumbar spine, i.e. increased lordosis of the lower lumbar spine so that the foot in the air can come down towards the ground. The amount of fixed flexion deformity of the hip joint can be assessed by Thomas test (Fig. 5.13). This test is done in the following sequence:

1. Patient lies supine on an examination couch with firm mattress (Fig. 5.14).

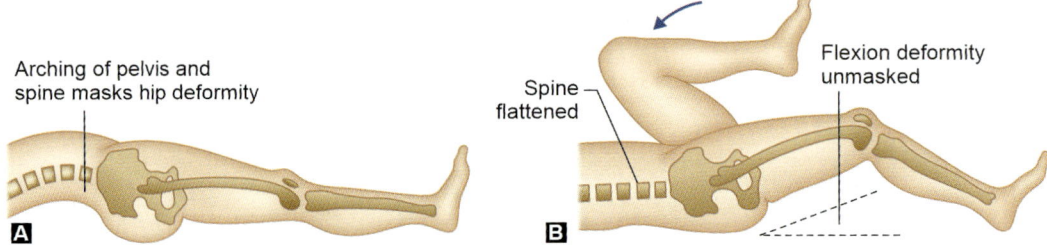

Arching of pelvis and spine masks hip deformity

Spine flattened

Flexion deformity unmasked

A   **B**

Fig. 5.13: Mechanism of Thomas test

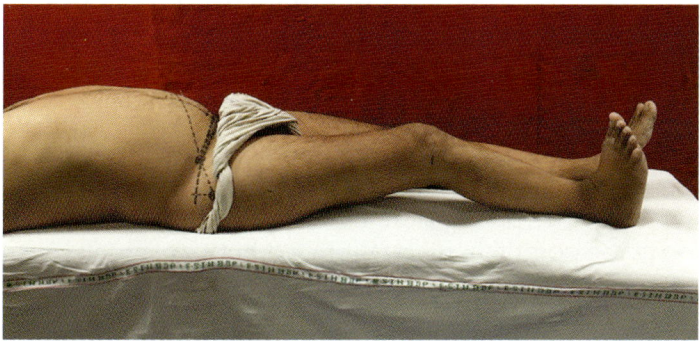

Fig. 5.14: Thomas test—patient lying supine on firm couch

2. The examiner insinuates his hand between the patients back and the couch to reconfirm the presence of increased lumbar lordosis. The dorsum of the insinuating hand is towards the back of the patient and palm towards the couch (Fig. 5.15).
3. The normal lower limb is acutely flexed at the hip and knee joint and then forced further to cause movements at the lower lumbar spine.
4. As the normal extremity, fully flexed at hip and knee, is further forced into flexion the lumbar lordosis corrects itself and the flexion deformity starts appearing at the diseased side (Fig. 5.16).

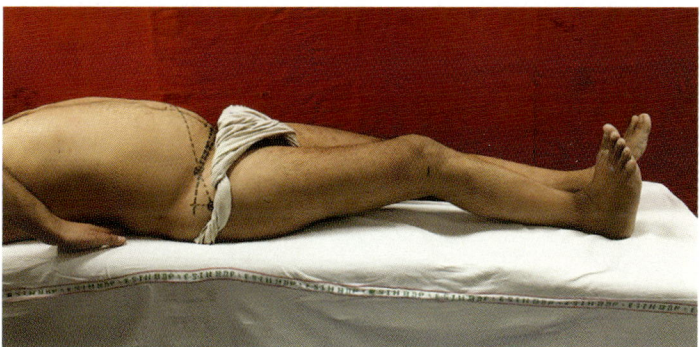

Fig. 5.15: Thomas test—checking for lumbar lordosis

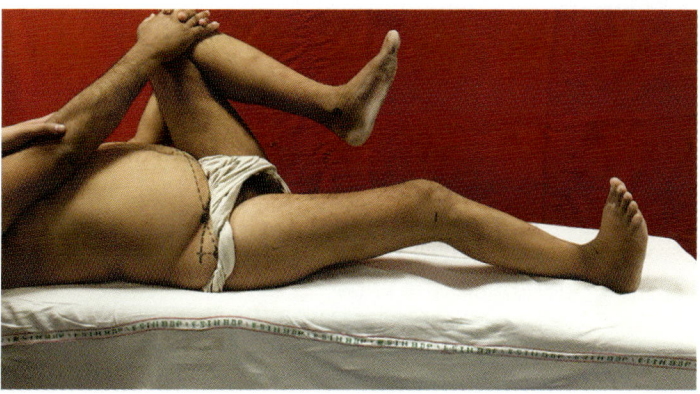

Fig. 5.16: Thomas test—acute flexion of normal limb

5. The forced flexion movements of the normal extremity is done to a point where lumbar lordosis is obliterated and the lumbar spine lies flat against the couch.

6. Holding the hyperflexed normal extremity in one hand the examiner lightly pushes on the anterior thigh of the diseased side which is now in flexion, to correct any excessive flexion of the diseased side beyond the genuine flexion deformity (Fig. 5.17). The gentle push of the hand on the anterior thigh of diseased side should stop at the point where the flattened lumbar spine again starts becoming lordotic (Fig. 5.18).

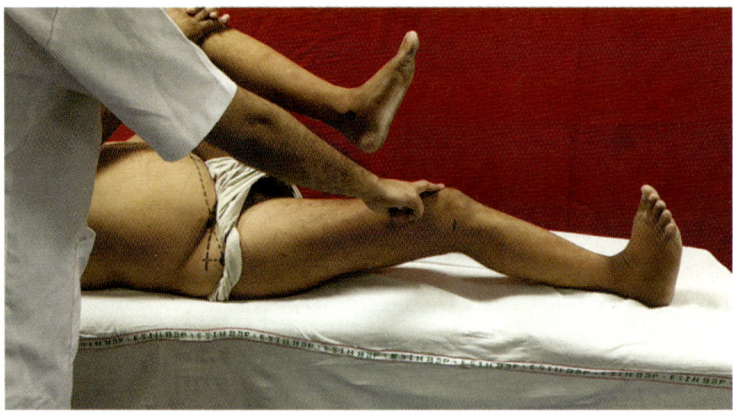

Fig. 5.17: Thomas test—correction of excessive flexion

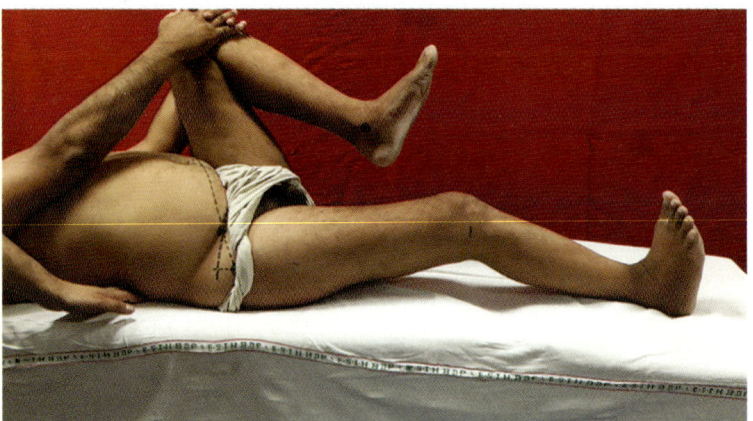

Fig. 5.18: Thomas test—obliteration of lumbar lordosis is checked

7. In this position, the angle made by the flexed diseased extremity with the couch is measured with the help of goniometer.

Note that the goniometer is kept at the base of the trochanter. The horizontal limb of the trochanter is kept parallel to the couch (Fig. 5.19).

Assessment of Bilateral Fixed Flexion Deformity

If both the hips of a patient are diseased and have flexion deformity, then patient has gross exaggeration of lumbar lordosis, which is contributed by both the hips.

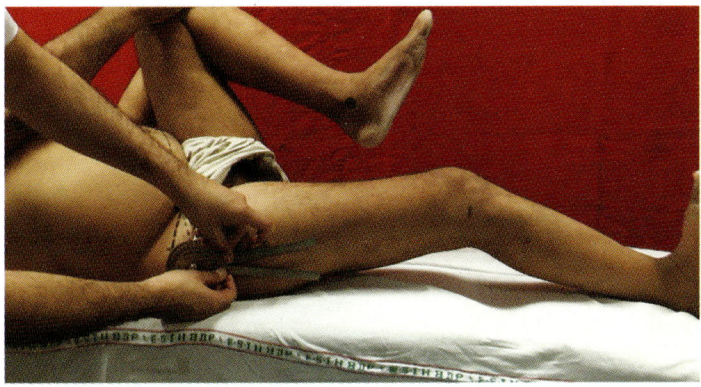

Fig. 5.19: Thomas test—measurement of fixed flexion deformity

Conventional Thomas test cannot accurately measure the flexion deformity of an individual hip in this situation. A prone test has been described in this situation.

Prone test for bilateral fixed flexion deformity of hip: The patient is made to lie prone on examination couch, in such a manner that pelvis is supported on the couch with hips at the edge of the couch. Both the lower limbs are hanging from the edge of the table in this position. Since both the hips are in flexion, this obliterates the lumbar lordosis caused by deformity in both the hips. Examiner places one hand over the pelvis to perceive any movement when the test is performed. With the other hand, examiner extends the hip to be tested, by holding and extending the thigh passively. In this way, the hip is extended passively till a resistance is felt and pelvis starts moving, which can be felt by the other hand of examiner placed on pelvis. At this point, the angle made by axis of the thigh and the axis of trunk is measured, which gives the amount of fixed flexion deformity of the hip on that side (Fig. 5.20).

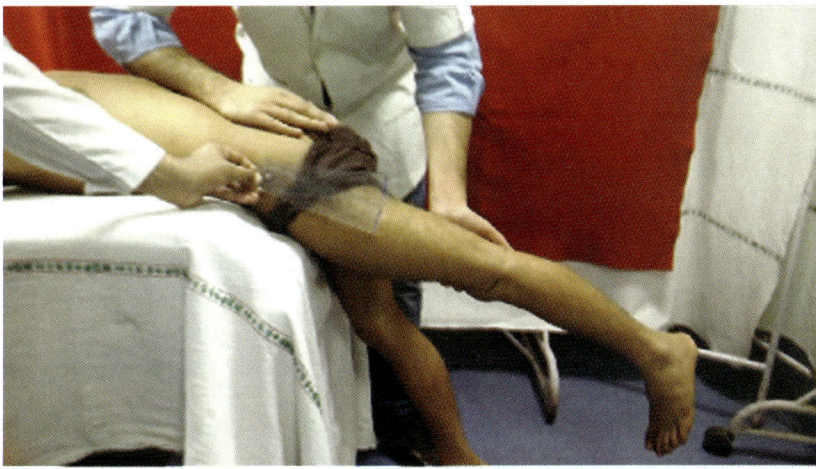

Fig. 5.20: Measurement of fixed flexion deformity (in bilateral hip involvement) using prone test

This test becomes impractical, if the patient is hefty or has difficulty in lying in prone position. It is applicable mostly in children.

The author has described a test which can be done in supine position: With patient in supine position, both the lower limbs are lifted and flexed passively at the hips till the time lumbar lordosis is obliterated. From the flexed position of the limbs, one limb is held in the same flexed angle, while the limb to be tested is gradually extended passively by the examiner to the point the pelvis just starts moving, i.e. lumbar lordosis starts appearing. The angle made between the couch and the partly flexed thigh under test gives the amount of fixed flexion deformity of the hip on that side (Fig. 5.21).

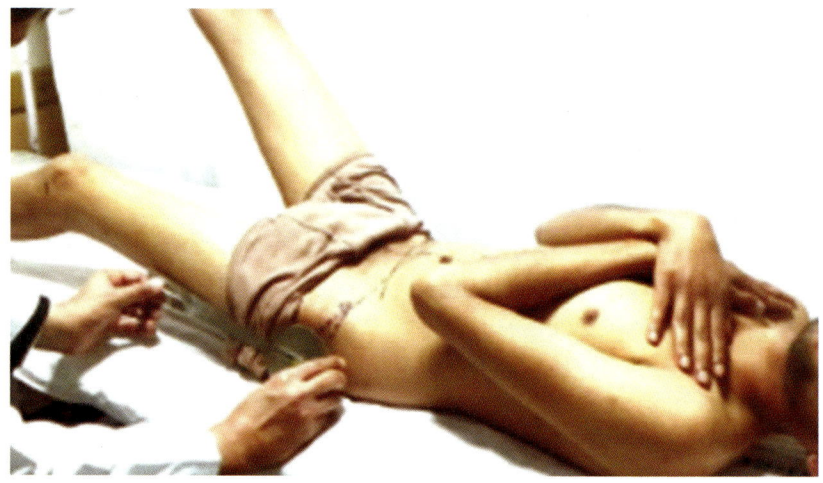

Fig. 5.21: Measurement of fixed flexion deformity (in bilateral hip involvement) with test done in supine position

Fixed Adduction and Abduction Deformity

The discrepancy in the level of two ASIS, noticed while inspecting the patient from front, conveys to the examiner, the possibility of the presence of fixed abduction/adduction deformity.

One should understand the mechanism of the difference in level of the two ASIS in frontal plane fixed deformity (abduction/adduction) of the hip joint.

In a case of uncompensated adduction deformity, where the hip joint is fixed in adduction, the limb and foot moves medially in the frontal plane and is off the ground. In this fixed position of the hip joint, the patient will not be able to ambulate. To make the ambulation possible, the foot is brought down from this adducted position to the ground by compensatory movements in the lower lumbar spine. The lower lumbar spine gets curved in the frontal plane, in a way that the concavity of the curve is towards the side of diseased limb and convexity towards contralateral side. This curvature in the lumbar spine leads to obliquity of the pelvis in a manner that the ipsilateral hemipelvis (consequently anterior superior iliac spine) is higher compared to the contralateral hemipelvis. The obliquity and the higher level of the hemipelvis on the ipsilateral side ensures that the adducted limb and foot moves from adducted position to a new position in a way that foot is plantigrade on the ground. Patient with fixed adduction deformity of the hip joint will thus be able to stand on both the feet and walk.

A similar mechanism occurs in a case of abduction deformity. On the affected side, when the hip is fixed is abduction, the limb and the foot on that side is in the air since it is lying lateral to the midline in the frontal axis. To bring the foot down to the ground, there is compensatory scoliotic movement of the lower lumbar spine in a manner that there is convexity towards the affected side and concavity of the curve towards contralateral side. The hemipelvis (ASIS) on the affected side moves down distally and the hemipelvis on the contralateral side moves up.

Measurement of Abduction and Adduction Deformity Steps

Measurement of Adduction Deformity (Fig. 5.22)

1. Patient lies supine on an examination couch with firm mattress.
2. The two anterior superior iliac spines are marked with a marking pen. In a patient of adduction deformity of the hip joint, the examiner can appreciate that on the affected side, the anterior superior iliac spine is on a higher level.
3. The examiner moves the affected limb to an adducted position, observing the change in level of anterior superior iliac spine. The raised anterior superior iliac spine starts coming down as the limb is adducted.

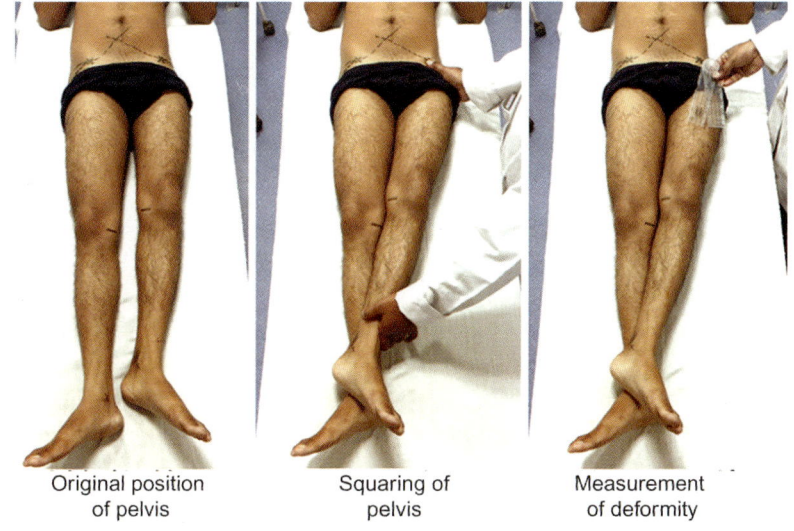

| Original position of pelvis | Squaring of pelvis | Measurement of deformity |

Fig. 5.22: Fixed adduction deformity

4. The affected side limb is adducted till the anterior superior iliac spine on the affected side comes to the same level as the contralateral anterior superior iliac spine, i.e. the two anterior superior iliac spines are at same level and pelvis is squared.
5. This manner of squaring the pelvis makes the compensated adduction deformity apparent.
6. The extent of deformity can be measured by either of the two methods:
   a. Angle between axis of limb and a line drawn through the ASIS in the sagittal plane, parallel to mid-sagittal plane.
   b. Angle between the two lines, one line joining the two ASIS in compensated position and the other line joining the two ASIS in uncompensated method (Kothari method).
      The first method is usually done in exam and exact amount is calculated with goniometer.

Measurement of Abduction Deformity (Fig. 5.23)

1. Patient lies supine on an examination couch with firm mattress.
2. The two anterior superior iliac spines are marked with a marking pen. In a patient of abduction deformity, the examiner can appreciate that on the affected side, the anterior superior iliac spine is on a lower level.
3. The examiner moves the affected limb to an abducted position observing the change in level of anterior superior iliac spine. The lower anterior superior iliac spine starts coming up as the limb is adducted.
4. The affected side limb is abducted till the anterior superior iliac spine on the affected side comes to the same level as the contralateral anterior superior iliac spine, i.e. the two anterior superior iliac spine are at same level and pelvis is squared.
5. This manner of squaring the pelvis makes the compensated abduction deformity apparent.

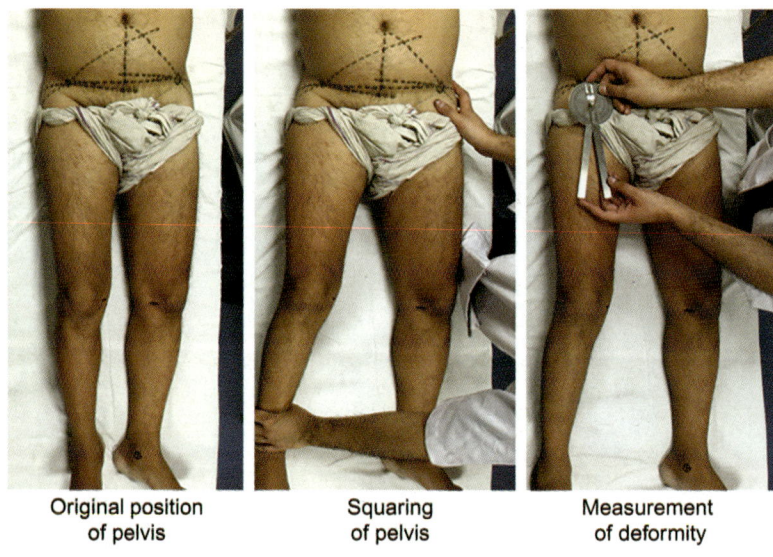

| Original position of pelvis | Squaring of pelvis | Measurement of deformity |

Fig. 5.23: Fixed abduction deformity

6. The extent of deformity can be measured by either of the two methods:
   a. Angle between axis of limb and a line drawn through the ASIS in the sagittal plane, parallel to mid-sagittal plane.
   b. Angle between two lines, one line joining the two ASIS in compensated position and the other line joining the two ASIS in uncompensated method (Kothari method).

The first method is usually done in exam and exact amount is calculated with goniometer.

Rotational Deformity (Fig. 5.24)

A diseased hip may also be fixed in a malrotation which can either be internal rotation or external rotation. The degree of rotation of the lower extremity is assessed indirectly by the position of the patella and direction of the toes. In normal anatomical position of the body, the patella and the toes are in approximately 10 (5–15)° of external rotation.

In a diseased hip, when the hip joint is fixed in increased external rotation, the patella and the toes come to lie in that much external rotation. Similarly if the diseased hip is fixed in internal rotation, the patella and the toes come to lie in internal rotation. Note that no compensatory mechanism are required when the hip is fixed in malrotation since the patient is able to ambulate whether the limb is in external rotation (Charlie Chaplin gait) or internal rotation (intoeing).

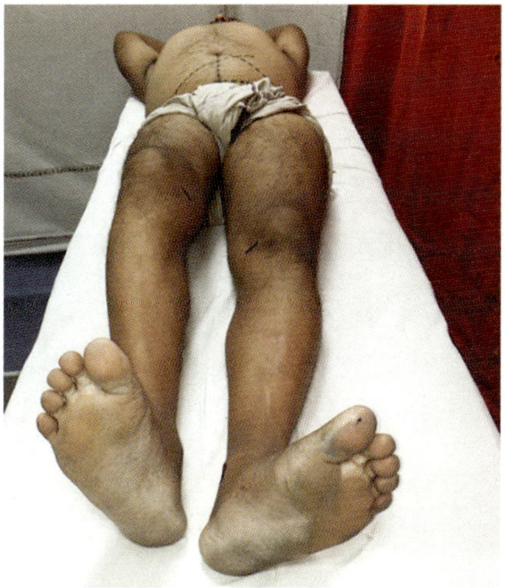

Assessment of Rotation Deformity

Patient lies supine on an examination couch, which has firm mattress.

Fig. 5.24: External rotation deformity on left side

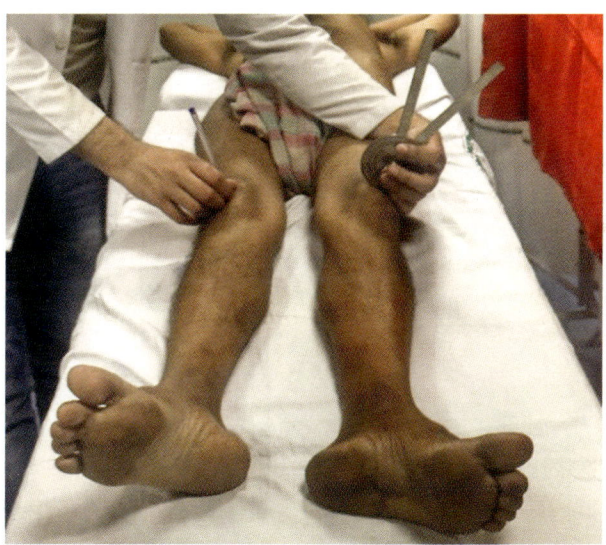

Fig. 5.25: Measurement of external rotation deformity

The amount of rotation deformity is assessed by drawing two lines through the patella as follows:
1. Through the centre of patella in the direction towards the roof in which the patella is pointing in the deformed position.
2. Other similar line when the patella is in the normal anatomical position.
   Angle is measured with the help of a goniometer kept at centre of patella (Fig. 5.25).

6

Movement, Measurements and Special Tests

+ Movement
+ Measurements

+ Special Tests

MOVEMENT

To determine any abnormality in the range of motion of a joint, examiner must know the normal range of movements in different directions of that joint. Being a ball and socket type of joint, hip joint has wide range of movements—flexion, extension, abduction, adduction and rotations (Table 6.1). Circumduction is a specific movement occurring at the hip joint. It is a combination of all the other movements. It is comparable to the movement of circumduction at shoulder. All the movements must be checked actively and passively. There may be a difference in active and passive movement, if the patient has a painful pathology or a muscle paralysis. For testing these movements, examiner must stabilize the pelvis first, and compare the movement with that of the normal hip in the same patient, as the range of each movement varies with individuals.

Table 6.1: Movements of hip joint	
Name of movement	Range
Flexion	0° to 90° (knee extended) 0° to 120° (knee flexed)
Extension	0° to 20°
Abduction	0° to 45°
Adduction	0° to 35°
Internal rotation	0° to 35°
External rotation	0° to 45°

Flexion

Flexion is tested in supine position, with back of thigh, calf and heel touching the bed. In extended knee, the hamstrings prevent the flexion of hip beyond 90°; while in a flexed knee, when the hamstrings are relaxed, further flexion up to 120° or till the anterior thigh touches the abdomen is possible (Figs 6.1 to 6.4).

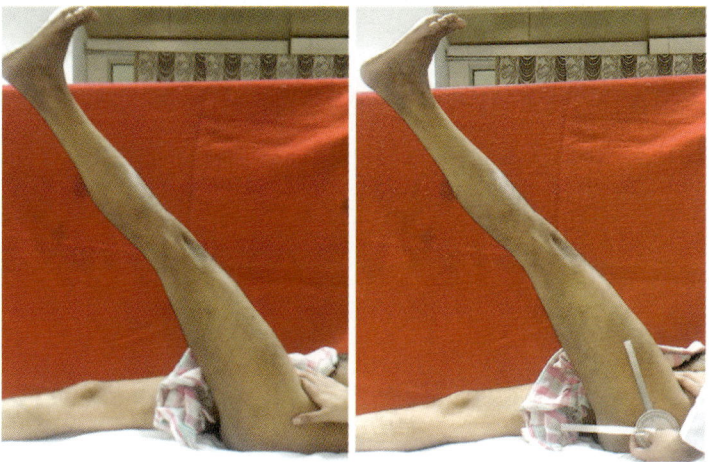

Fig. 6.1: Flexion with knee extended—active movement

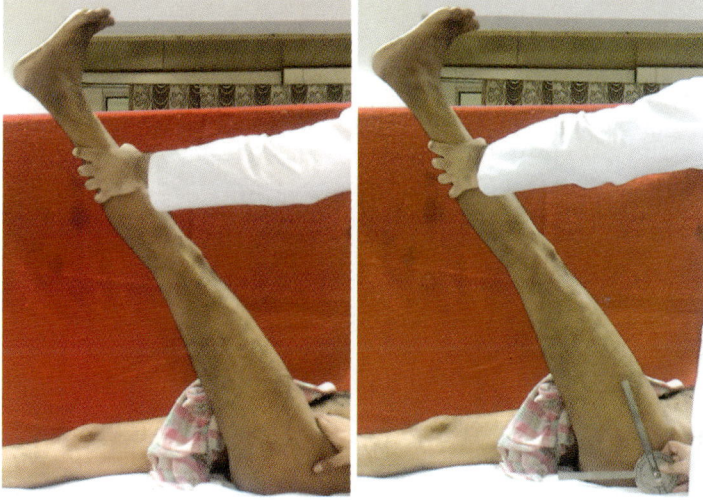

Fig. 6.2: Flexion with knee extended—passive movement

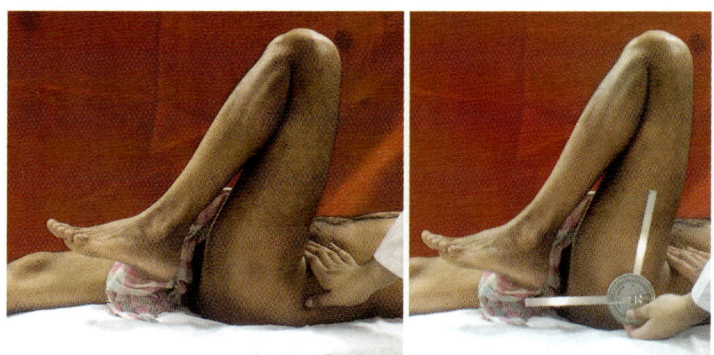

Fig. 6.3: Flexion with knee flexed—active movement

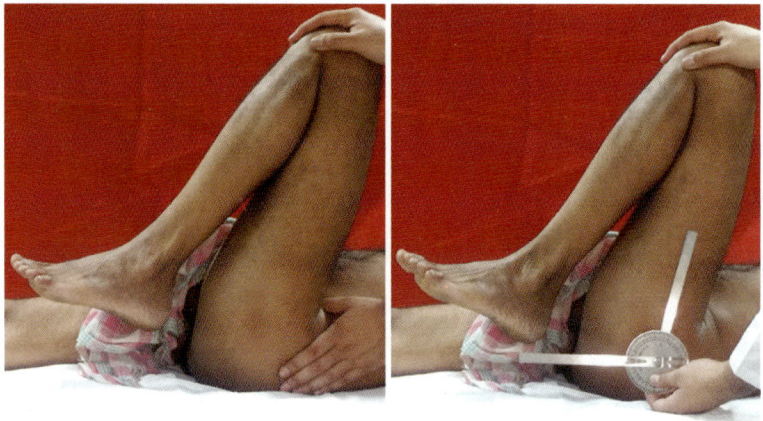

Fig. 6.4: Flexion with knee flexed—passive movement

Measurement of Movement of Flexion in a Hip Fixed in Flexion Deformity

In a hip joint which has a fixed flexion deformity, the movement of extension is absent, but further range of flexion may be present. This range of free flexion is assessed by the following method.

The Thomas test to determine the flexion deformity is carried out as explained previously. From the position till which the flexion deformity is visible and measured in the Thomas test, further range of flexion movement is assessed by the examiner passively. The examiner grasps the flexed thigh from the position of its deformity and gently moves it towards further flexion. This movement of further flexion is continued till a point after which the pelvis starts moving. The movements of the pelvis are examined by the other hand of the examiner which grasps the pelvis.

The final statement regarding the range of flexion movement in hip joint with fixed flexion deformity may read as follows: Right hip joint has a fixed flexion deformity of 40°, further flexion is possible from 40–80° and flexion from 80–120° (normal ROM) is absent.

Extension

Extension is best tested by asking the patient to lie prone on the table. The patient is then instructed to lift the extremity with the knee extended, this is done passively also. It is possible up to 20°. Loss of extension is the first sign of effusion of the hip joint.

Abduction

To test abduction and adduction, the long axis of both the limbs and that of the trunk should be parallel to each other, so far as possible. The patient is instructed to move the limb laterally in direction of abduction. The limb is abducted to a point where the pelvis starts moving, the angle between the original position of limb and that of the abducted limb is measured with the help of goniometer. Normal range of abduction is 0–40°. The same test is done passively by the examiner who keeps one hand on the same side hemipelvis, and with the other hand grasps the limb at the ankle and moves it in direction of abduction till the pelvis starts moving. Any difference in the active and passive ROM is noted.

Adduction

After fixing the pelvis and placing his hand over anterior superior iliac spine, the examiner holds the leg at the ankle in his other hand and moves it medially to access passive adduction. If an assistant is present, the opposite limb is lifted to allow the limb being tested to be adducted while in full extension. If assistant is not available, cross the limb being examined over the other limb which is touching the mattress. The limb is moved medially till the point when the pelvis starts moving. The start of the movement of the pelvis is accessed by the examiner's hand grasping the anterior superior iliac supine.

In case an adduction deformity is present, abduction movement will be absent. However, further adduction may be present. To access this further adduction, following sequence is adopted (Fig. 6.5).

1. Pelvis is squared by adducting the affected side.
2. Adduction deformity is assessed.
3. Keeping one hand on the hemipelvis of the affected side, the limb is further adducted from the already adducted position.
4. The adduction manoeuvre is continued till the hemipelvis just starts moving (perceived by examiner's hand on the hemipelvis).
5. The new position of the limb gives the final adduction movement.

The active adduction is tested by asking the patient to adduct the limb actively, till the point, the pelvis starts moving.

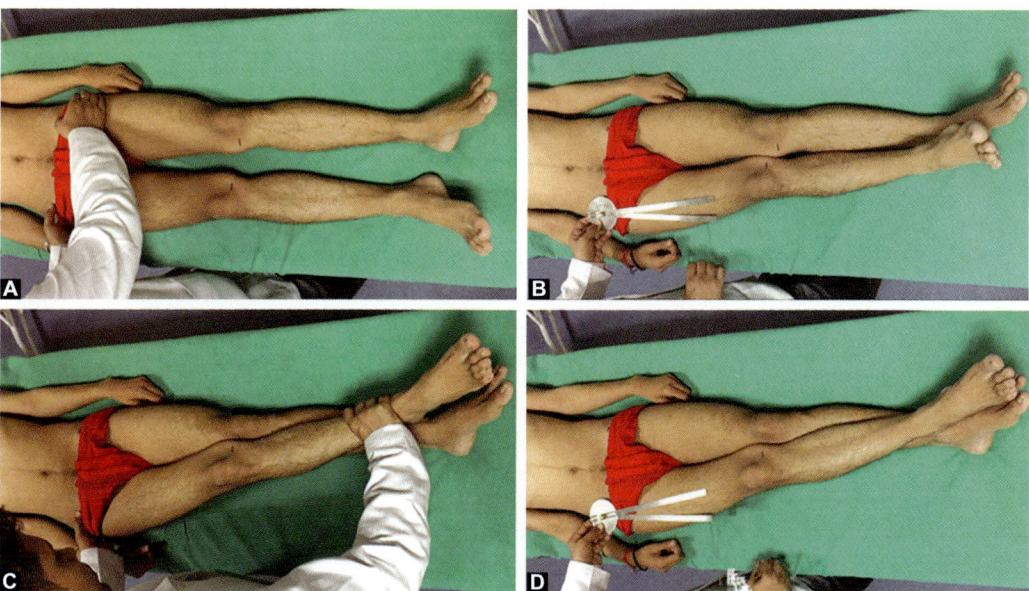

Fig. 6.5A to D: Assessing free adduction beyond adduction deformity: (A) Rt. ASIS higher—adduction deformity; (B) Pelvis squared, adduction deformity—15°; (C) Further adduction possible; (D) Final adduction 30°, free adduction 15 to 30°

Rotations

Internal and external rotations can be tested either in extended position of hip or in 90° flexion of hip joint.
- In extended position, rotation can be assessed by placing hand over thigh and rotating the limb. The foot is observed as an index of degree of rotation possible.
- In 90° flexion of hip, the knee is held with one hand and the foot is moved laterally to assess internal rotation, and medially to assess external rotation. It is important to note here, that when foot moves laterally or externally, the hip rotates internally and vice versa. Normal range of external and internal rotation is 0–45° in this position.

Drehmann Sign, Sectoral Sign, Movement Axis Deviation, Femoral Acetabular Impingement

Drehmann sign was described by Gustav Drehmann in 1904. He described this test for patients of old slipped capital femoral epiphysis (SCFE). In this sign, an unavoidable passive external rotation of the hip occurs when performing hip flexion. In addition, internal rotation of the affected hip joint is restricted/not possible/painful (Fig. 6.6).

Procedure: The patient is lying supine and with the flexed knee, the hip is passively flexed. The hip flexion falls short of 90° or so in neutral position of the hip (Fig. 6.7). It appears as if hip flexion is reduced. However, further flexion of the hip is possible when the hip is slightly abducted and external rotated.

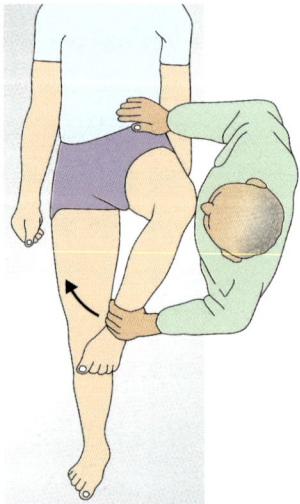

Fig. 6.6: Drehmann sign

A detailed study by Makoto Kamegaya et al in 2011 has conclusively proved that it is because of cam-type femoroacetabular impingement, which follows the slipped upper femoral epiphysis displacing posteroinferiorly. (Drehmann sign and femoroacetabular impingement in SCFE, Pediatr Orthop, Volume 31, Number 8, December 2011.)

A similar sign, attributed to Whitman (1909), has been mentioned in the literature. (Richolt JA, Teschner M, Everett PC, Millis MB, Kikinis R. Impingement simulation of the hip in SCFE using 3D models. Comput Aided Surg 1999; 4:144–151)

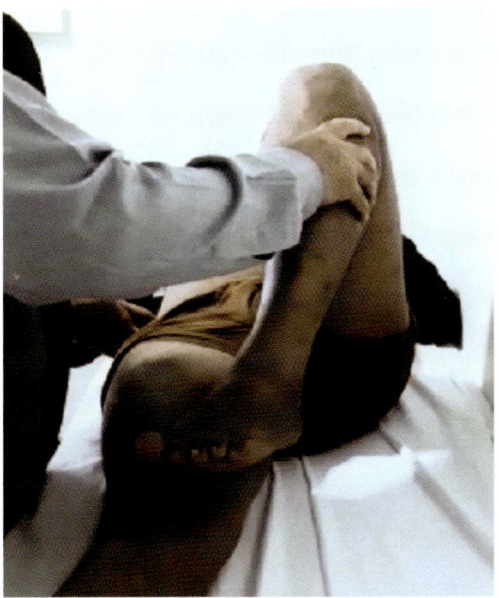

Fig. 6.7: Hip flexion stops at 90° in neutral hip position

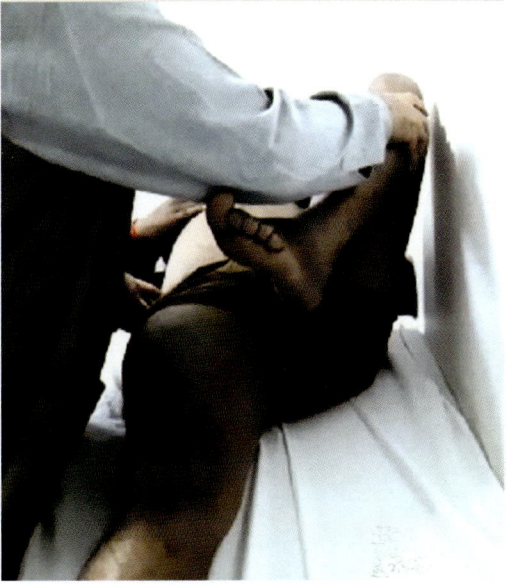

Fig. 6.8: Full hip flexion possible in abduction and external rotation

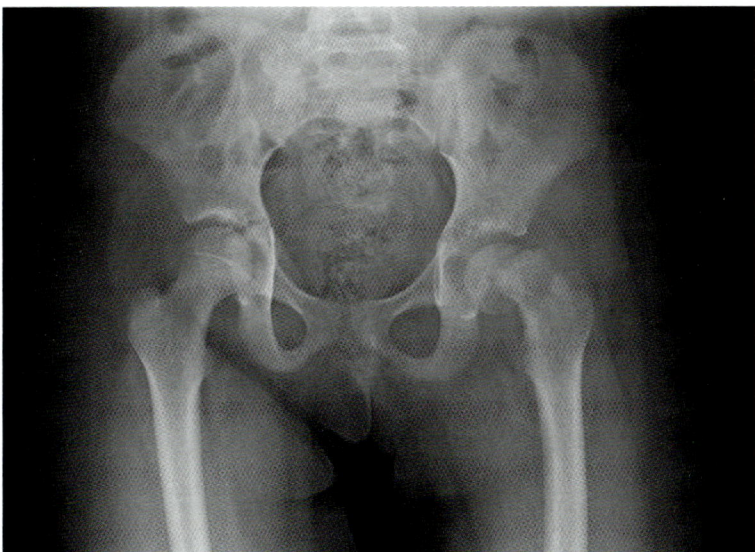

Fig. 6.9: Slipped capital femoral epiphysis—X-ray

Axis deviation in hip movements: The fact of complete hip flexion possible only on abduction and external rotation (Fig. 6.8) in patients of old SCFE (Fig. 6.9) and other similar situations of femoroacetabular impingement, like in AVN, osteoarthritis of the hip, lead to a situation where on full flexion of the hip, the knee is pointing towards the ipsilateral shoulder, instead of the normal situation of pointing towards contralateral shoulder. This has been described as axis deviation of hip (movements).

A **Sectoral sign**, which is similar, has been described in patients suffering from avascular necrosis of the head of the femur. In this, the range of internal rotation is less in hip flexion, compared to when the hip is in extension. It has been named so, believing that a specific involved area or sector of femoral head causes obstruction, in flexed hip when internal rotation is attempted. When the hip is in extension, an uninvolved or normal area of the femoral head articulates on attempted internal rotation which is then possible without hindrance.

MEASUREMENTS

Different physical dimensions are:
1. Limb length
   a. Apparent length
   b. True length
2. Supratrochanteric shortening
3. Girth
4. Anteversion of neck

Limb Length

Apparent Length

The lower extremity has a peculiar situation where, the apparent length or the visual impression of the length may not be same as the actual or real length of the limb. This is because of two reasons:
1. The length of the extremity is assessed proximally from the anterior superior iliac spine and not from the centre of the head of the femur, which lies deep and not palpable. As a result, if the pelvis changes its position from its normal horizontal status, i.e. becomes oblique, the length of the limb (as taken from ASIS) changes on visual impression.
2. The peculiar mechanism of compensation required in frontal plane deformities (abduction/adduction) to achieve ambulation. There is pelvic obliquity as compensation, which takes the hemipelvis (ASIS), either proximally or distally, depending upon whether there is adduction or abduction deformity.

One must appreciate that in the situation of fixed abduction deformity, the hemipelvis (ASIS) moves down and there is apparent lengthening, while in adduction deformity, the hemipelvis (ASIS) moves up and there is apparent shortening.

It is not an uncommon situation in a patient of hip disease with fixed abduction deformity, where there is apparent lengthening and at the same time actual (real) shortening. Obviously the apparent length of the limb is measured in the position of the limb in which the patient presents, while the real length is measured by making the fixed frontal plane deformity obvious.

Galeazzi's test (Allis sign): It is a quick visual method, which was described by Allis to observe difference in lengths of the two lower limbs. If the two lower extremities are kept in a position of hip at 60° flexion and knee at 90° flexion, so that the feet touch the couch in side-to-side position, one can check the level of limb length discrepancy by the level of knees. There will be a difference of level of knees in case of limb length discrepancy. On the side in which the limb is short, the knee will be at a lower level (Fig. 6.10). The level of knee would also be different not only in the height but in a proximal and distal direction also, depending upon whether the shortening is in the femoral or in tibial component. In an instance where the femur is short, the knee on that side would not only be lower, it would also be proximal (Fig. 6.11). While in another instance, where the lower limb is short because of tibial shortening, the affected side knee joint would be lower and distal.

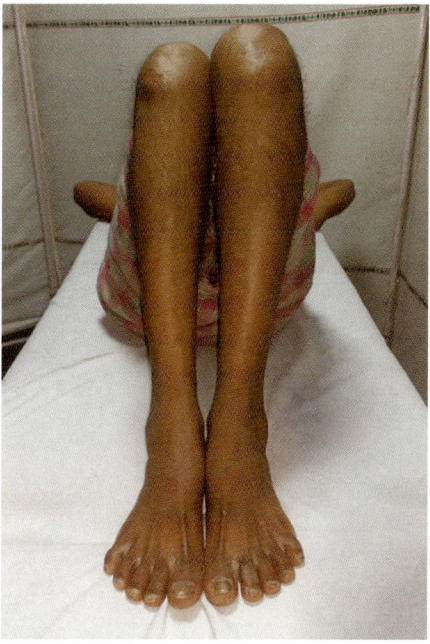

Fig. 6.10: Shortening of right lower limb

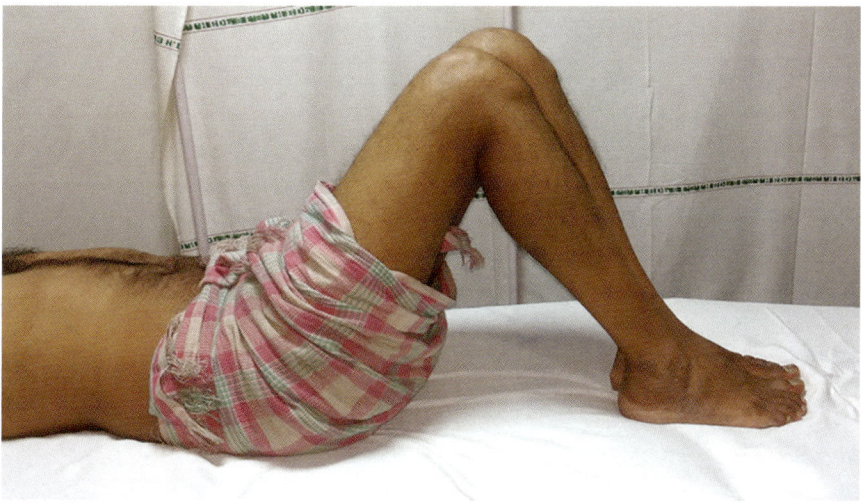

Fig. 6.11: Allis test—showing shortening of right lower limb due to femoral component (right knee is lower and proximal)

Measurement of limb length: Before initiating the step of measurements, following points should be marked with a marker pen:

1. ASIS
2. A fixed point on the medial side of the knee, which is either joint line or adductor tubercle.
3. Tip of medial malleolus

The limb length is measured in two segments, femoral segment from the ASIS to the fixed medial point at the knee, and leg length from medial fixed point to tip of medial malleolus.

Measurement of apparent length: Patient lies supine on a couch with firm mattress in whatever position, the limbs are lying. The limbs should be 'parallel', so much as possible. The apparent length of the extremity is measured between any fixed point in midline of body, i.e. sternum, xiphisternum, pubic symphysis or umbilicus (a bony fixed point is preferable) to the tip of medial malleolus (Figs 6.12 and 6.13).

With the lower limbs lying parallel to each other, the apparent length of the normal and affected limb is taken and recorded (Figs 6.12 and 6.13).

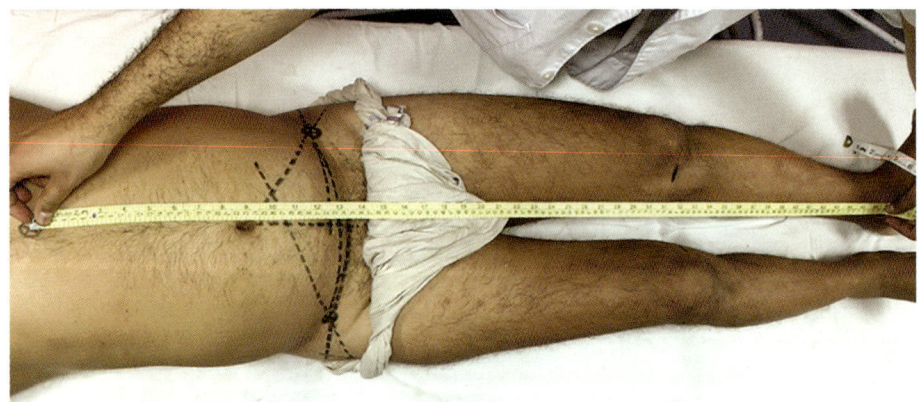

Fig. 6.12: Measurement of apparent length of normal limb

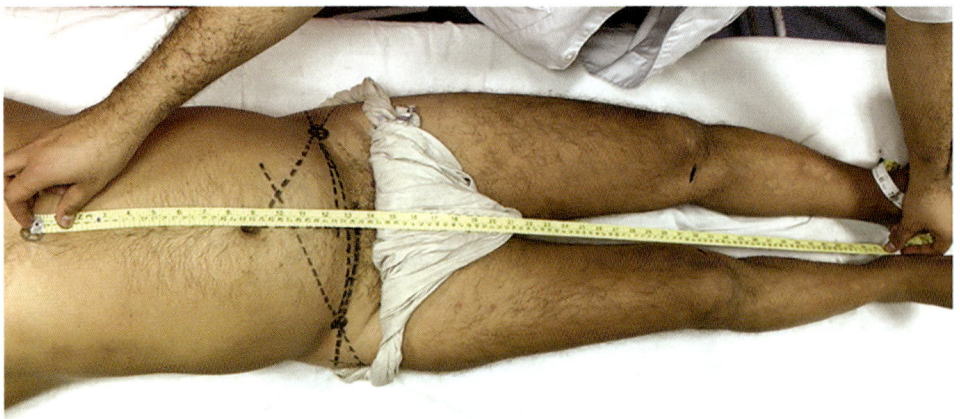

Fig. 6.13: Measurement of apparent length of affected limb

Measurement of True Length

As a prerequisite for this measurement, the frontal plane deformity of the limb, i.e. abduction and adduction are revealed by bringing the affected limb into the position of deformity. The limb length is then measured. For proper comparison, the normal limb is taken into the same position of abduction/adduction and the measurements taken on that side.

In adduction deformity

1. The examiner holds the affected side limb at lower part of leg with one hand and takes the limb gradually into adduction, while with the other hand kept on the ilium, the movements of pelvis are perceived. In a patient of fixed adduction deformity, as the limb is moved into adduction, the previously raised ASIS starts coming down. The limb is taken gradually into increasing degrees of adduction till the two ASIS are at the same level, i.e. pelvis is squared. The limb length is then measured from the previously marked points, i.e. ASIS, medial knee point, medial malleolus.

2. The normal limb is then kept in an equal amount of adduction. The length of the normal limb is then measured, preferably in two segments.

A practical tip: In a case of severe adduction deformity exceeding 15–20°, as the affected side limb is moved to adduction, it will cross the normal limb in a scissor fashion with the normal limb lying along the mattress and the adducted affected limb crossing over it. While measuring the length of the normal limb in corresponding degree of adduction, the positions of the limbs should be changed suitably—the affected adducted should be in contact with the mattress and the normal limb should cross over it.

In abduction deformity (Figs 6.14 and 6.15)

1. With one hand, the examiner holds the affected limb at the lower part of the leg and takes it gradually into abduction, while with the other hand kept on the ilium, the movements of pelvis are perceived. As the amount of abduction is increased, the previously lower ASIS raises in level. Abduction is continued till both anterior superior iliac spines are at the same level, i.e. pelvis is squared. The length of the limb is then measured in two segments.

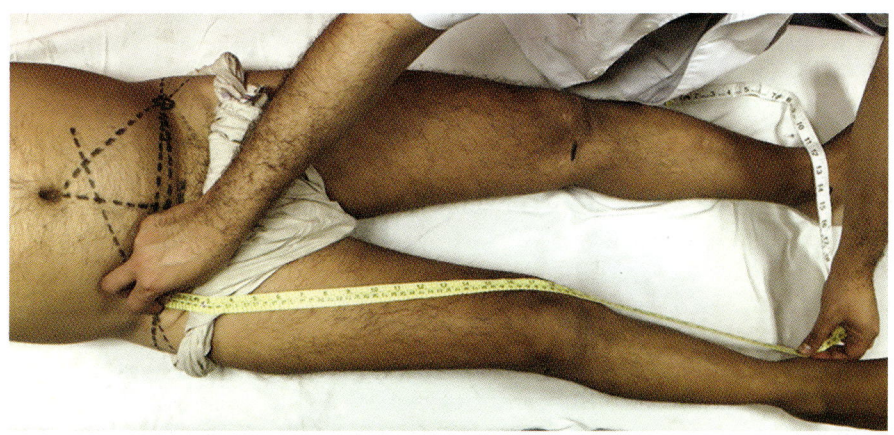

Fig. 6.14: Measurement of true length of affected limb after squaring of pelvis

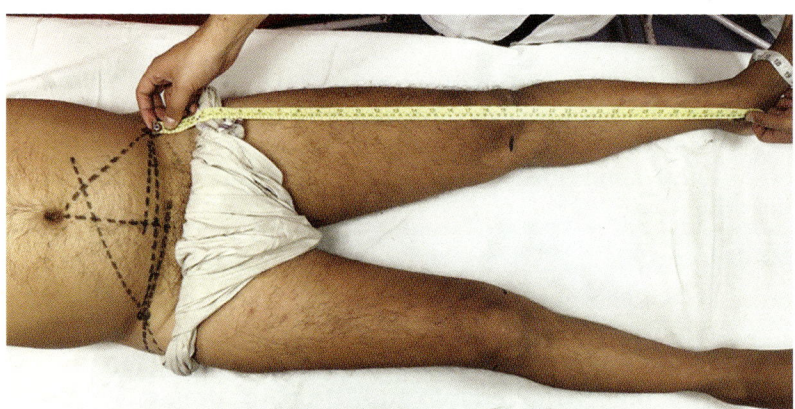

Fig. 6.15: Measurement of true length of normal limb—kept in same degree of abduction as affected limb

2. The normal limb is then kept in an equal amount of abduction, while the pelvis is squared and the affected side limb is lying in the previously achieved abduction. The length of the limb is measured preferably in two segments.

Supratrochanteric Shortening

Femur has got two distinct segments—a segment above trochanter and a segment below trochanter. It is important to find out whether the discrepancy in length of the two sides is in supratrochanteric segment, infratrochanteric segment or both. This knowledge, of where exactly is the shortening, helps not only in arriving at a diagnosis but also in subsequent management.

Different methods have been described to assess supratrochanteric length of femur and any shortening in it:
- a. Bryant's triangle
- b. Nelaton's line
- c. Shoemaker's line
- d. Chiene's line

Bryant's Triangle (Described by Thomas Bryant)

To draw this triangle, three points are marked:
- i. Tip of greater trochanter
- ii. Anterior superior iliac spine
- iii. The third point lies at the junction of two lines—one line is a perpendicular drawn from the ASIS to the couch and the other line is along the longitudinal axis of shaft of the femur drawn proximally. A point where these two lines meet is marked.

The triangle is drawn by combining these three points (Fig. 6.16). The length of the base of this triangle denotes the supratrochanteric length of the femur. When the length of the base of the triangle is compared on two sides, it gives an idea of the proximal migration of the greater trochanter and supratrochanteric shortening. In a case of destruction of the hip joint or fracture of the neck of the femur, the base will be smaller and consequently patient would be having a supratrochanteric shortening.

Note: The term supratrochanteric length does not correspond to the length of the neck of the femur. It is a descriptive term, used to signify proximal migration of greater trochanter. The length of the neck in real terms cannot be measured clinically.

Bryant's triangle can also give an idea about the inward migration of the head of femur—like in protusio acetabuli, central fracture dislocation of hip. The length of the side of the Bryant triangle joining the tip of greater trochanter and the anterior superior iliac spine will be reduced in case of inward migration of head of femur (Fig. 6.16).

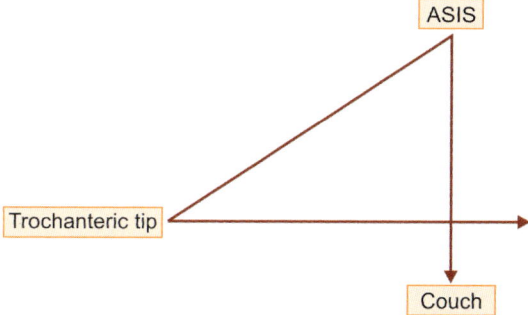

Fig. 6.16: Bryant's triangle

Nelaton's Line (Fig. 6.17)

This is a *qualitative* method to measure or observe the proximal migration of the trochanter, the exact migration cannot be measured in absolute amount.

Test is done in the following manner:

Patient lies in the lateral position. The limb which is away from the couch and towards the examiner is flexed to 90° at hip and knee. The limb is then allowed to drop and rest on the couch in this flexed position of hip and knee. A line is then drawn from the anterior superior iliac spine to the most prominent part of ischial tuberosity. The tip of greater trochanter is then marked. In normal circumstances, the tip of greater trochanter would just be touching the line joining ASIS with ischial tuberosity.

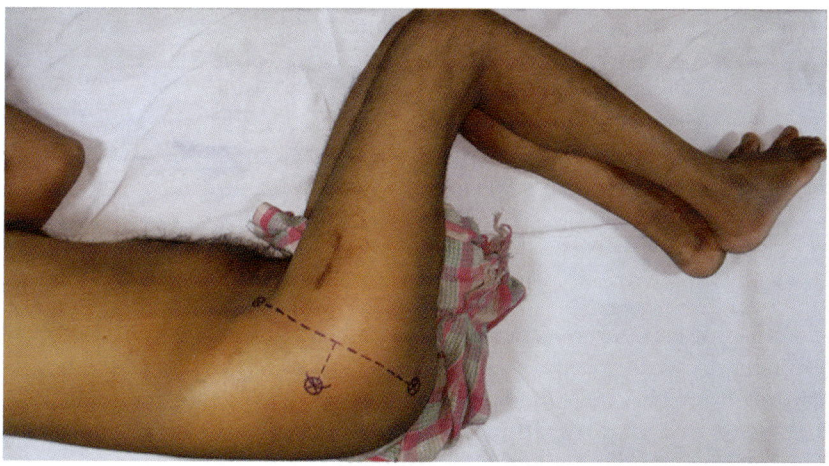

Fig. 6.17: Nelaton's line showing proximal migration of trochanter

In case of supratrochanteric shortening, the tip of greater trochanter is migrated proximally beyond this line.

It is not possible to measure the exact supratrochanteric shortening by this method. This test has the advantage of being independent of the other hip since the two sides are not being compared. However, this test cannot be carried out in a situation, where because of disease, hip and knee cannot be flexed to 90°. In that situation, the two sides should be compared in an identical position of hip and knee flexion to get an idea of proximal migration of trochanter—hip and knee are flexed to the extent possible and the position of the trochanter in relation to the line joining the anterior superior iliac spine and the ischial tuberosity is noted. Then, on the normal side, the same observation is done by keeping the normal hip and knee in identical degree of flexion.

Shoemaker's Line (Fig. 6.18)

This again is a qualitative test.

With the patient lying supine, a line joining the tip of greater trochanter to the anterior superior iliac spine is prolonged towards the anterior abdominal wall. A similar line is drawn on other side.

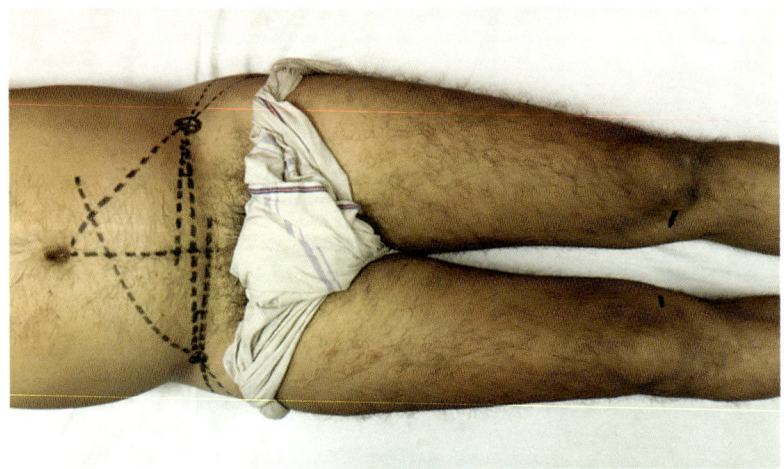

Fig. 6.18: Shoemaker's line

Normally these lines meet in the midline at or above umbilicus.

In cases of supratrochanteric shortening, these lines meet below the umbilicus. The meeting point will also be not in midline but would be on the normal side, opposite to the side of proximal migration of greater trochanter.

Chiene's Lines (Fig. 6.19)

In supine position of patient, a Chiene's line/parallelogram is drawn joining the two ASIS. Another imaginary line, joining the tips of the trochanter is drawn. (A scale or a similar straight tool can be kept to denote this line.) These two lines are normally parallel. In case of proximal migration of greater trochanter on one side, the lines no longer remain parallel and converge on that side.

A few clinicians like to describe it as a Chiene's parallelogram.

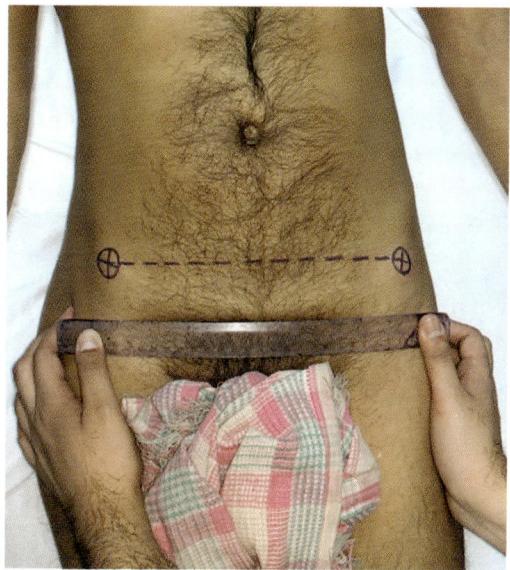

Fig. 6.19: Chiene's line

Girth

The observation of the wasting made during inspection and palpation can be quantified by measuring the circumference of the thigh and the leg. This measurement should be done at the most muscular part at the identical points on the two sides. For example, about 5 inches from base of trochanter at thigh and about 4 inches from tip of fibular head along the calf.

Anteversion of Neck

The amount of version in head and neck segment of femur is usually not done in all cases. It is of specific importance in those cases in which the previous clinical examination has indicated altered version, e.g. presence of in-toeing or out-toeing, excessive internal rotation with correspondingly reduced external rotation, etc., however, it is a sound policy to measure the angle of version in each case by Craig's test (Ryder method).

Craig's Test/Ryder's Method

In cases of suspected excessive anteversion or retroversion of the femoral neck, Craig's test can be done to assess the anteversion of the femoral neck. Excessive anteversion would be indicated by intoeing of the feet and retroversion by out-toeing (Charlie Chaplin gait).

It is done by the following method:
1. Patient is made to lie prone on the table.
2. The two limbs are checked one by one.
3. On the side to be checked, knee is flexed to 90° with the hip in neutral flexion/extension.
4. Holding the foot and ankle in one hand (knee flex 90°), the limb is rotated internally and externally while other hand of the examiner palpates the trochanter.

5. The limb is held in the position where the trochanter is maximally prominent or felt is noted.
6. In the above position of rotation (trochanter is maximally prominent), the angle formed between the long axis of tibia (in the flexed knee) and the midline is measured. This is the angle of anteversion of the femur (Fig. 6.20).

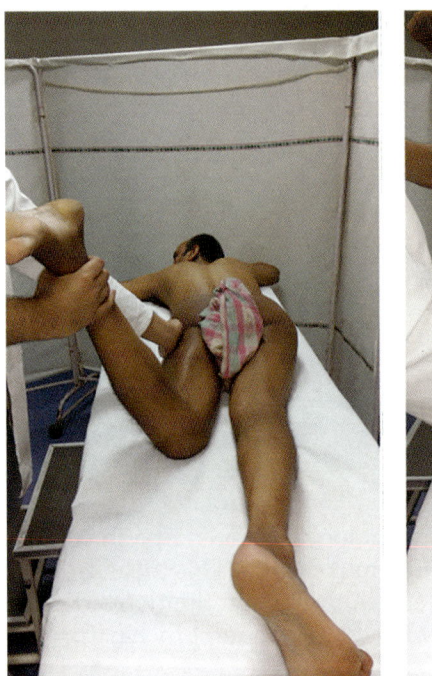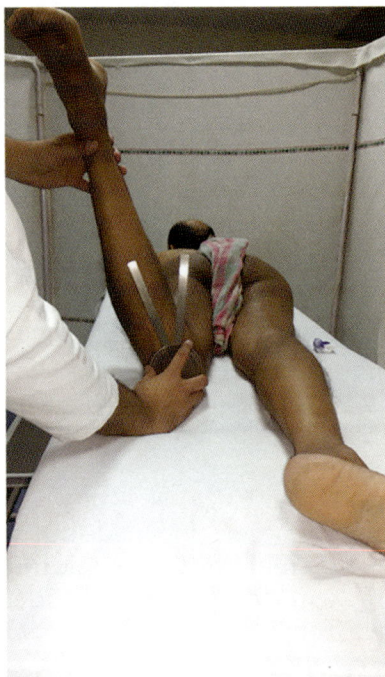

Fig. 6.20: Measurement of anteversion

The logic behind this test is that trochanter is most prominent when the neck is parallel to the floor, i.e. anteversion has been negated. This anteversion is negated by internal rotation of the femur. The required anteversion of the femur is indirectly indicated by the position of the tibia. The test has its limitations in the sense, that it cannot be carried out if the patient cannot lie prone, rotations of the femur are absent or the knee cannot be flexed to 90°.

SPECIAL TESTS

Trendelenburg Test (Fig. 6.21)

It is a test to determine the integrity of abductor mechanism of the hip joint in single leg stance, i.e. if the patient is standing on the right lower limb, the abductor mechanism of the right side is being tested. The abductor mechanism of the hip is a first-degree lever with hip joint as the fulcrum which has weight of the hemipelvis of unsupported limb on one-side and abductor muscles as force on the other side. One should understand, that the abductors of hip, which in stance phase, counteract the weight of the other side limb and pelvis which is unsupported, for example—abductor muscles of left side (when left side is in stance phase) counteract the weight of the right side hemipelvis

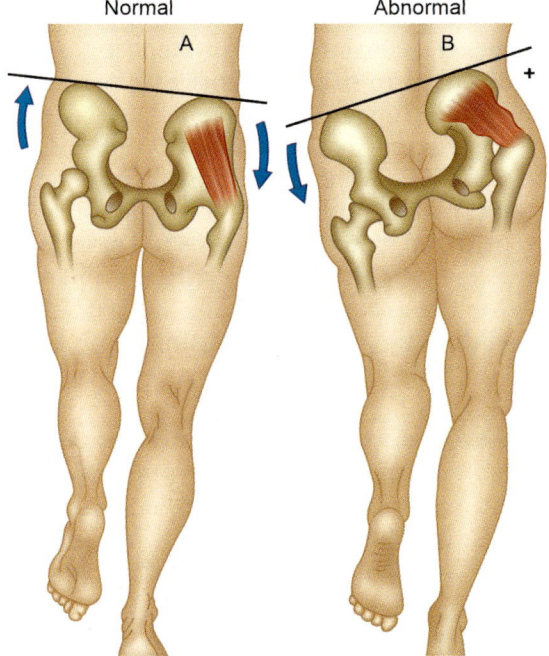

Normal   Abnormal

Fig. 6.21: Trendelenburg test

which is unsupported. As a prerequisite, Tredelenburg test can be done in those patients who are cooperative and are able to stand in single leg stance on the diseased limb for 30 seconds. The test is done in the following manner:

1. The examiner stands behind the patient to conduct this test.
2. The level of posterior superior iliac spines, gluteal folds and the trunk in general (marked by level of scapula and shoulder joints) are observed.
3. The patient is asked to lift one leg, and to stand and bear weight on the other leg which is being tested. Preferably the patient should fold the arms across the chest while doing this.
4. The change in level of the previously marked PSIS and gluteal fold of the side, which is in air, is observed.
5. In a normal person, these two points (PSIS and gluteal fold) either rise or remain at the same level, i.e. there is no fall.
6. In a case of positive test, the posterior superior iliac spine and the gluteal fold tend to fall on this side (which is in the air and non-weight bearing).
7. In an effort to counteract this fall, patient tries to bend the trunk towards the weight-bearing side ,which results in fall of level of shoulder tip and scapula on this side ,which is weight bearing.

Sometimes the test is not positive in the initial few seconds, but becomes positive after some time, i.e. delayed Trendelenburg test. It is seen in situations where the patient has good normal trunk musculature.

Assisted Trendelenburg Test

If the patient is not able to stand on the affected leg without support, then the examiner can assist the patient in bearing weight. This is called assisted Tredelenburg test and

is done in the following manner:
1. The examiner stretches out his hands, while standing in front of the patient.
2. The patient is encouraged to take support by placing his/her palms on the outstretched hands of the clinician.
3. First the patient is instructed to bear weight on the normal side, while taking support of the hands of the examiner. The clinician assesses the amount of pressure exerted by the patient on his hands. It will be equal on both sides.
4. The patient is now asked to stand on the affected side, while taking the support of the clinician's outstretched hands. If the patient's left side is diseased and he is attempting to stand on this side, while taking support of clinician's outstretched hands, he would feel that the patient is exerting more pressure on the left hand. Patient's right hand is used to put more pressure on the left outstretched hand of clinician (Fig. 6.21).

Similarly if the patient has got a diseased right hip joint and is attempting to stand on this side, while taking the support of clinician's outstretched hand, the patient will put more pressure on clinician's right hand. The patient would use his left hand to put more pressure on clinician's right hand.

Trendelenburg test will be disturbed, if any part of the abductor mechanism is affected, i.e.
1. Fulcrum—hip arthritis, avascular necrosis of head of femur.
2. Lever arm disturbance—fracture neck of femur, coxa vara, coxa valga
3. Force disturbances, i.e. disease of abductor muscles—post polio residual paralysis, muscle dystrophy, etc.

Telescopic Test (Fig. 6.22)

This test is performed to assess containment of the femoral head in the acetabulum. It is a passive test and conveys stability of the hip joint.

It is done in the following manner:
1. Patient lies supine on the examination couch.
2. The examiner passively flexes the affected hip and knee of the patient to 90°.

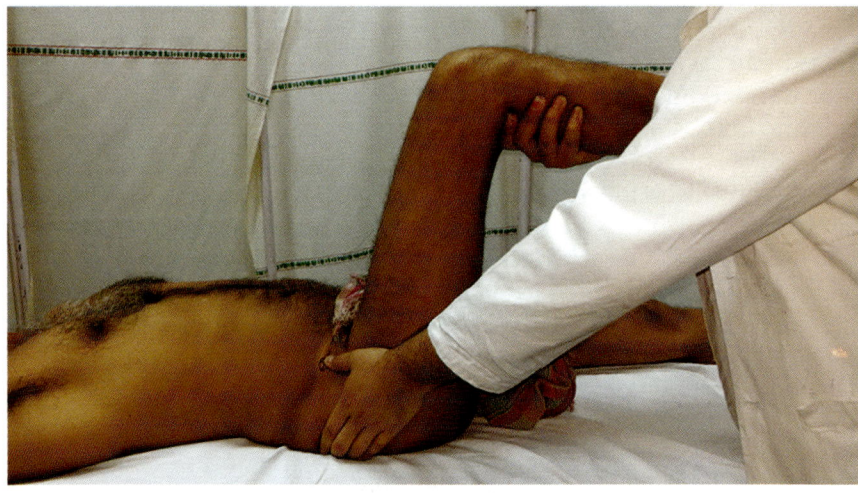

Fig. 6.22: Telescoping test

3. The examiner then holds the lower thigh of patient with one hand, letting the leg of the patient rest on his own forearm.
4. The examiner applies a pull and push force with his hand holding the patient's thigh. The examiner keeps his other hand on the gluteal area just proximal to the trochanter.
5. The examiner assesses any abnormal mobility by excessive downward and upwards movements of the trochanter.
6. The hand of the examiner, which is kept in the gluteal area proximal to the trochanter, would feel the excessive mobility of the trochanter.
7. A bony round swelling, conforming to the shape of femoral head and moving excessively with pull and push movements, can be felt in a case of dislocated hip (congenital or traumatic).

Craig's Test

This test is used to check for anteversion of the femoral neck. Please refer to page 65 for details.

Tests to Measure Contractures around the Hip

A few tests are done only when they are specifically indicated:
1. **Pseudo-flexion deformity in iliopsoas muscle spasm:** In a case of psoas abscess (usually tubercular in origin) or any other irritating focus in the vicinity, there is iliopsoas muscle spasm and contracture which causes flexion deformity of the hip joint named pseudo-flexion deformity. This flexion deformity is in contrast to the true flexion deformity of the hip joint seen in hip joint diseases. The two can be distinguished in the following manner.
   In a patient who has got a pseudo-flexion deformity of the hip joint because of iliopsoas muscle spasm, if the hip is taken into 90° flexion, rotations of the hip joint are free and without pain. Any attempted extension would, however, elicit severe pain. In contrast, in a case of a hip joint disease causing flexion deformity of the hip, the rotations will be painful and restricted in flexed hip also.
2. **Ober's test:** This is to rule out contracture of the tensor fascia lata muscle and of the fascia lata, resulting in flexion contracture of the hip joint. It results not only in flexion of hip but some amount of associated abduction and external rotation also. The test is done in the following manner:
   a. The patient lies in the lateral position with the affected side up.
   b. The examiner holds the leg, acutely flexes the hip and the knee and then abducts the limb.
   c. The limb, acutely flexed at hip and knee and abducted at hip, is left in the air and the manner of fall of the limb is observed. In case there is contracture of the fascia lata, the limb is held in the air for some time before it falls, which it will do gradually. While in absence of tensor fascia lata contracture, it falls freely and immediately.
      A modified Ober's test has also been described. In this test, the limb acutely flexed at hip and knee and abducted, is extended at the knee before it is allowed to fall. Again the manner of the fall is observed.
3. **Ely's test:** This test has been described to measure contracture of rectus femoris muscle, particularly reflected head.

Patient lies prone on the bed. With the knee held in 90° flexion, the examiner passively extends the hip joint. The other hand of the examiner is kept on the area of sacrum. In case the rectus femoris contracture is present, patient's buttock and the pelvis are lifted off the couch.

Examination of the hip joint is incomplete without examination of the following:
- Opposite hip joint
- Both knee joints
- Spine particularly sacroiliac joint
- Distal neurovascular deficit
- Per rectal examination to look for ischiorectal abscess and central dislocation of hip.

For common tests for sacroiliac joint refer to book *Orthopaedic Clinics—Spine* by Sudhir K Kapoor.

7

Angular Deformities of Hip

(Coxa Vara and Valga, Anteversion and Retroversion)

+ Neck-shaft angle
+ Coxa vara
+ Coxa valga

+ Torsional configuration of upper end of femur and its deviations

---

Femur has got two distinct segments:

1. Shaft—with condyles at one end and trochanter at the other end
2. Neck and head segment.

These two segments join in a peculiar manner—they join at an angle to each other in the coronal plane which is called *neck-shaft angle*. At the same time, the planes of the two segments are in a different rotational orientation, i.e. version of the femoral head and neck.

This angular and rotational orientation of the two segments is poorly understood by many. The purpose of this chapter is to explain the fundamentals of this orientation and at the same time outline the clinical significance of this.

NECK-SHAFT ANGLE

The axis of the neck and the head segment is at an angle to the long axis of the femoral shaft, which is called *neck-shaft angle*. This angle can be measured accurately in an anteroposterior radiograph of the hip joint. Two lines are drawn—one line passing through mid-axis of femur shaft, and another line passing along mid-axis of femoral neck and the centre of the head. The angle between these two lines is the neck-shaft angle. It is also known as '*Mikulicz angle*'or '*caput-collum-diaphyseal (CCD) angle*' (Fig. 7.1).

Neck-shaft angle is 140–150° at birth and as the child starts bearing weight, it gradually reduces, to 120 to 135°. This is the result of differential muscle forces acting at this junction of the two segments. If

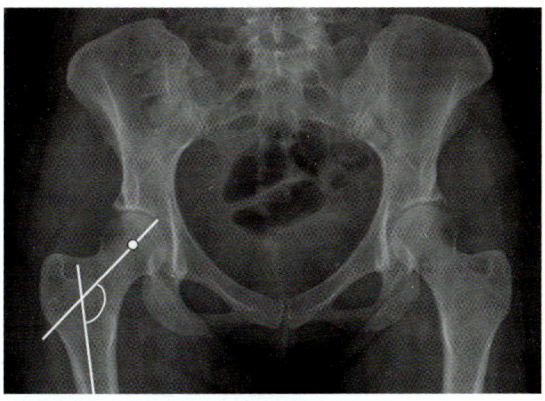

Fig. 7.1: Neck-shaft angle

the angle is less than normal, i.e. less than 120°, it is called *coxa vara* and more than 135°, it is called *coxa valga*.

◤ COXA VARA

The coxa vara could either be congenital, developmental or acquired.

i. **Congenital coxa vara:** It is found in association with other congenital abnormalities of the hip and femur like DDH, proximal focal femoral deficiency, etc. Sometimes, other congenital problems may also be present elsewhere in the body, like cliedocranial dysostosis, CACP (camptodactyly-arthropathy-coxa vara-pericarditis) syndrome.

This coxa vara is usually severe, femoral neck may be short and deformed and the head of the femur may be misshapen. The coxa vara is appreciated, when the parents bring the child with complaints pertaining to other congenital abnormalities.

ii. **Developmental (infantile) coxa vara:** This is the most common presentation of coxa vara per se. Child on presentation is between 2 and 6 years of age and the presenting complaints are painless limp and shortening.

The exact aetiology is not known, though the frequent finding is defective ossification in the medial and inferior part of the neck as seen on the X-ray (Fig. 7.2). In about one-third of the cases, it is bilateral.

On examination, the child has Trendelenburg or waddling gait (depending upon unilateral or bilateral disease), trochanter is proximally migrated, 1.5–2 cm of true supratrochanteric shortening, restriction of abduction and internal rotation, and positive Trendelenburg sign.

X-ray confirms the diagnosis of decreased neck-shaft angle. An inverted-shaped radiolucency in the inferior neck, on AP radiograph, is typical. A characteristic X-ray finding, beside the decreased neck-shaft angle, is beaking of the trochanter, i.e. trochanter tip takes the shape of a beak (Fig. 7.2).

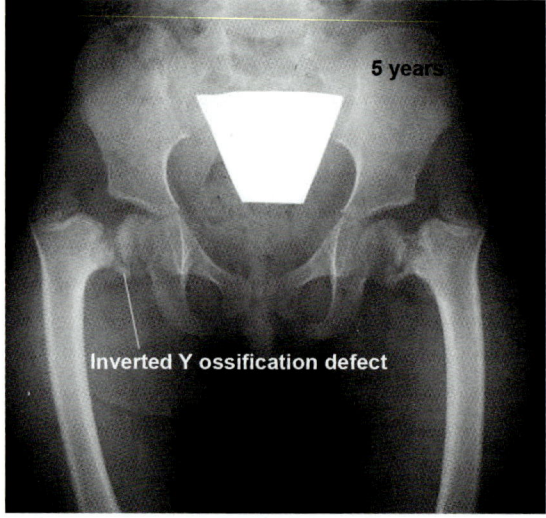

Fig. 7.2: AP X-ray of pelvis showing 'beaking of the trochanter'

The severity of the coxa vara is graded by Hilgenreiner's epiphyseal angle (Fig. 7.3), which is determined on anteroposterior radiograph, as an angle between Hilgenreiner's line and a line through the proximal femoral epiphyseal plate.

- Less than 25°—normal
- 25°–45°—mild, needs observation, may correct by itself
- 45°–60°—moderate, needs strict follow up, if progressive surgery.
- >60°—severe, needs surgery.

There is an associated decreased anteversion of the neck with this type of coxa vara. Surgery done for the correction of this deformity is a precise derotation, wedge intertrochanteric osteotomy.

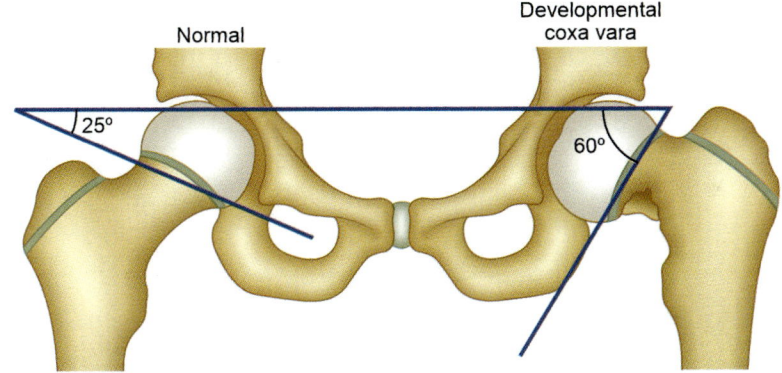

Fig. 7.3: Hilgenreiner's epiphyseal angle

iii. **Adolescent coxa vara:** This usually refers to the coxa vara following slipped capital femoral epiphysis. It is a gradually progressive problem. Refer to page no. 88.

iv. **Acquired:**
   a. *Post-traumatic:* This follows a fracture mostly in trochanteric area, which malunites in coxa vara. A traumatic slip of the upper femoral epiphysis may also lead to this.
   b. *Post-rachitic:* It follows poor mineralization in the physis, subsequent to vitamin D deficiency, and in association with other bony deformities which occur following active rickets.
   c. *Post-infective:* In a country which is endemic for tuberculosis coxa vara may occur following tuberculosis of the hip. Pyogenic osteomyelitis and septic arthritis may also lead to coxa vara.
   d. *Miscellaneous* like metaphyseal dysplasias, osteogenesis imperfecta, fibrous dysplasia, achondroplasia, Paget's disease, etc.

COXA VALGA

When the neck shaft angle is more than 140°, it is called coxa valga.

Coxa valga is usually a secondary condition and develops mostly following unequal muscle forces acting across the upper end of the femur.

Congenital variety, though known, is rare.

The common causes, which lead to abnormal muscle forces acting across the upper end of femur and consequently coxa valga, are:
- Spastic cerebral palsy
- Post polio residual paralysis
- Meningomyelocoele, etc.

Besides the situations of disturbed muscular balance around the upper end of femur, coxa valga may be seen in few dysplasias, e.g. Turner's syndrome. Premature differential closure of the growth plate following trauma, infection, surgical intervention may also cause coxa valga.

Coxa valga is often associated with increased femoral anteversion.

Clinical presentation depends upon the primary condition leading to coxa valga.

Diagnosis is evident on plain X-ray (Fig. 7.4).

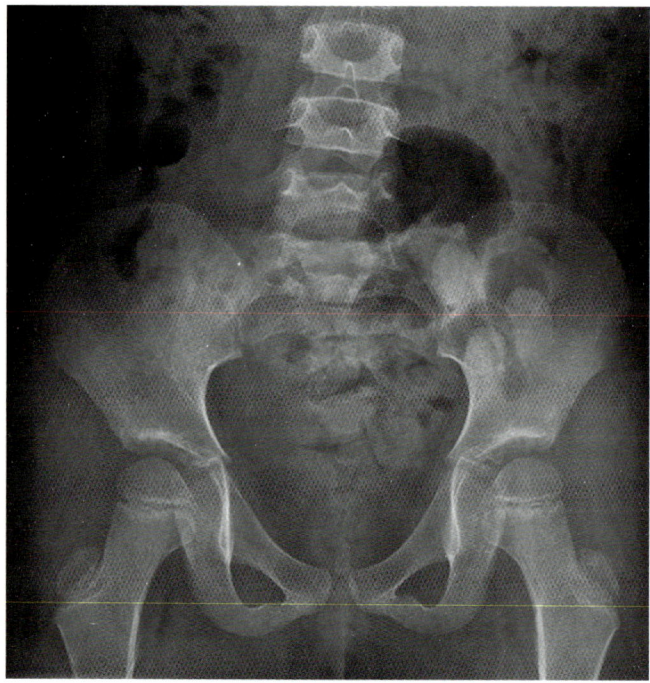

Fig. 7.4: Coxa valga

Treatment depends upon the acetabular coverage and development. If the acetabulum is well formed and providing adequate coverage to the femoral head, surgery is not indicated. However, if acetabulum is not providing good coverage, i.e. there is lateral subluxation head of the femur, surgery is indicated. An intertrochanteric derotation wedge osteotomy is sufficient. A preoperative X-ray in abduction, which shows a good femoral head coverage, is the prerequisite before the surgery.

TORSIONAL CONFIGURATION OF UPPER END OF FEMUR AND ITS DEVIATIONS

The two major long bones of the lower limb, femur and tibia, are rotated about their longitudinal axes. The normally present rotation is called 'version'. If the rotation becomes altered, either in magnitude or in direction, it is named 'torsion'. The amount of normal version lies within a range, rather than a fixed figure.

This version/rotation of a long bone can be determined by the angle between the axes of the proximal and distal ends. In case of femur, it is the angle between the axis of the head and neck segment and the axis of the condyles of the femur at the most posterior point, i.e. posterior condylar axis (Fig. 7.5).

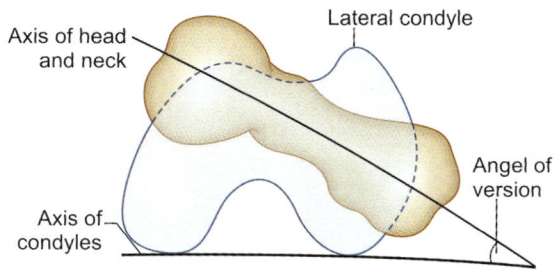

Fig. 7.5: Anteversion of neck (Image showing femoral neck superimposed on femoral condyles)

This concept has to be properly grasped that the frontal plane of the head and neck segment of the femur is at a rotational angle to the coronal plane of the shaft of the femur or the intercondylar plane of femur. Holding a femur bone end on helps (Fig. 7.6).

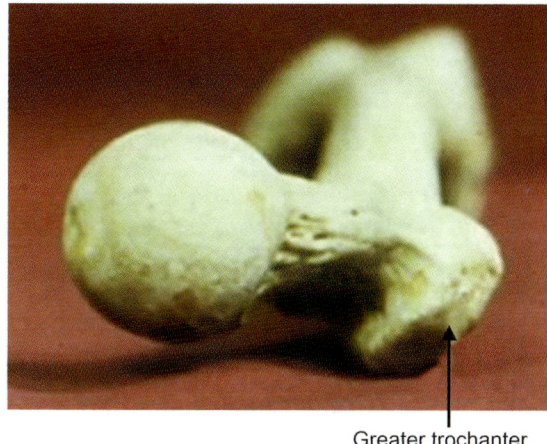

Greater trochanter

Fig. 7.6: Anteversion of head and neck (anatomical specimen)

The amount of version at birth is 30–40°, which decreases to the normal adult value of 10–15° by the age of 8 years. After the age of 8 years, hardly any further change occurs.

Clinical Presentation of Increased Version

Excessive anteversion is manifested clinically by intoeing gait, the so-called *pigeon gait*. Other causes of intoeing in children are metatarsus adductus and internal tibial torsion. Different causes at various ages are as follows:
1. Up to 1 year—metatarsus adductus—forefoot is adducted at tarsometatarsal joint and the hind foot is normal.
2. 1–3 years—internal tibial torsion
3. After 3 years of age—increased anteversion of the femur

The parents presenting the child till the age of 8 years, with the complaints of intoeing, should be reassured that it is likely to correct by 8 years of age.

If the troublesome intoeing, cosmetic or functionally, persists after the age of 8 years, it needs a further workup to know the cause and the amount of abnormality.

When anteversion is suspected, the following aspects are significant to delineate the problem.

1. **Position of the patellae:** In standing anatomical position, normally patellae point forward, while in case of intoeing, the patellae are facing medially (Fig. 7.7).

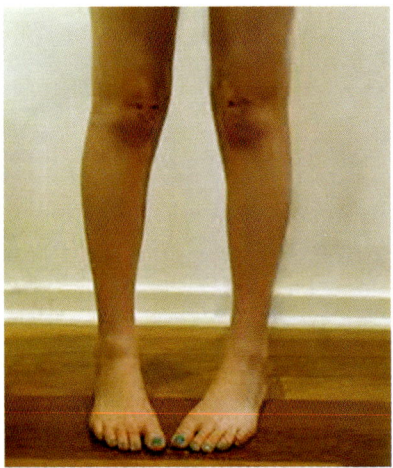

Fig. 7.7: Patellae are facing medially

2. **Foot progression angle (FPA):** This is the angle formed between the longitudinal axis of the foot and the line of progression, as the child walks (Fig. 7.8). Normally the FPA is around 10° (range—3 to 20°). In case of intoeing due to increased femoral anteversion, it is less than 3°.

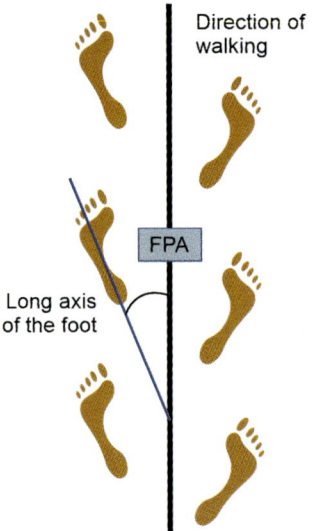

Fig. 7.8: Foot progression angle (FPA)

3. **Range of internal/external rotation:** In case of increased anteversion of the femur, internal rotation is increased and external rotation is correspondingly decreased. This arc and range of rotation is examined with the child in prone position and knee at 90° of flexion. The degree of anteversion can be graded in the following manner:

Grade of excessive anteversion	Internal rotation	External rotation
Mild	70–80°	10–20°
Moderate	80–90°	0–10°
Severe	More than 90°	Limb cannot be brought to neutral

The range of internal/external rotation are estimated in prone position with a knee flexed to 90°. The excessive internal rotation, subsequent to increased anteversion of the femur in the neck, is responsible for 'W' position adopted by these children, while sitting on floor.

Clinically the amount of femoral anteversion can be determined by performing Craig's test (refer to page 63). Plain radiographs (AP and lateral) of the pelvis with both hips cannot estimate the amount of anteversion. An apparent coxa valga, visible on the anteroposterior view, points towards increased anteversion. A few radiographic techniques have been described to measure femoral anteversion on plain X–ray, but these require special positioning techniques and conversion tables, which are not practical for routine clinical assessment.

Fluoroscopy can be helpful to quantify anteversion. The hip is rotated under fluoroscopy until a true AP view of the hip is obtained. The amount of internal rotation of the leg in that position is the femoral anteversion.

It is worthwhile to understand the significant aspects of two other diseases which commonly cause intoeing, i.e. metatarsus adductus and internal tibial torsion.

Metatarsus adductus	Internal tibial torsion
Physiological up to 1 year of age	Physiological up to 3 years of age
Assessment is done by "heel bisector line test" (Fig. 7.9). Normally the heel bisector line passes between the second and third toes. Grades of the deformity: ✗ **Mild:** Heel bisector line passes through the 3rd toe. ✗ **Moderate:** Line through 3rd and 4th toe web space. ✗ **Severe:** Line through 4th and 5th toe web space.	Assessment is done by: (i) **Thigh foot angle:** Patient is examined in prone position with the knee flexed to 90°. Two lines are drawn, one along the mid-axis of the thigh and the other along the mid-axis of foot. The angle between the two represents the amount of tibial rotation (Fig. 7.10). (ii) Examine patient in sitting position. Drop a plumb line from tibial tuberosity.
Treatment: If persists after 1 year of age, manipulation and serial casting. If persists late, surgery may be required.	**Treatment:** Mostly conservative. Very rarely surgical correction is required.

CT scan is the preferred method to detect femoral neck anteversion.

Decreased anteversion can lead to out-toeing (Charlie Chaplin gait).

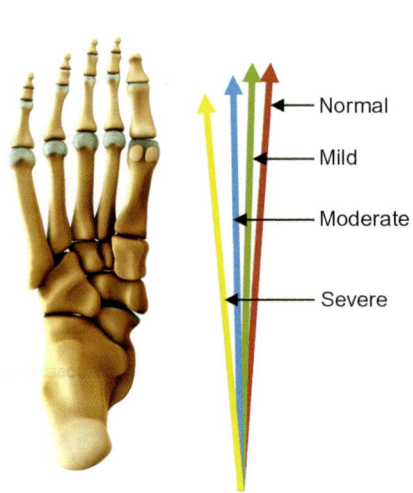
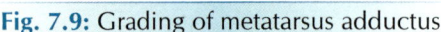

Fig. 7.9: Grading of metatarsus adductus

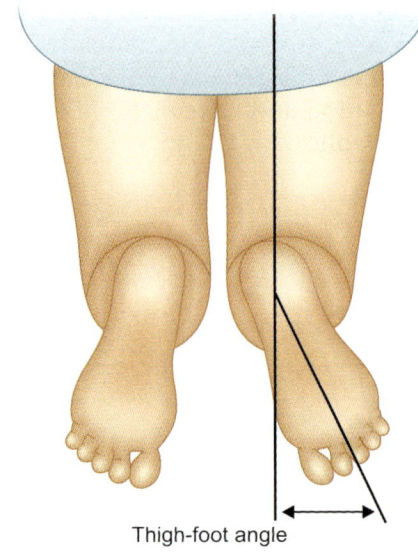

Fig. 7.10: Thigh-foot angle

Femoral Retroversion

When the normal angle of anteversion at the upper end of femur (10 to 15°) is reduced, it is named 'retroversion'. 'True or literal retroversion', i.e. the plane of the femoral head and neck section is rotated backwards in comparison to the coronal plane of the shaft, is rare. It may occur in cases of severe deformation of upper end of the femur by diseases like septic arthritis, dysplasias, etc.

The patient clinically presents with 'out-toeing gait' also nicknamed as 'duck gait' or 'Charlie Chaplin gait' (Fig. 7.11). On examination, external rotation of the femur is increased while the internal rotation is correspondingly decreased.

Most of the cases, which present in childhood, are automatically corrected by the adolescent age. Surgical correction is rarely required.

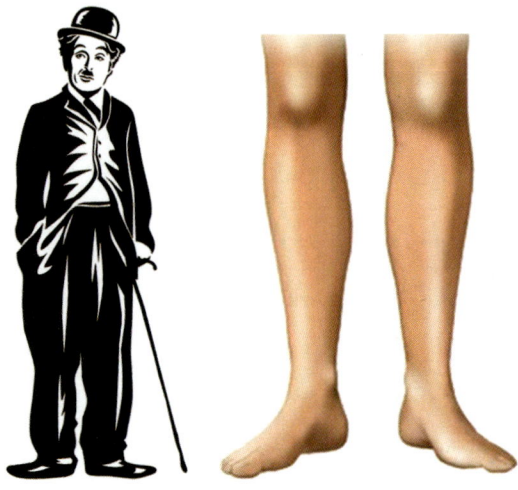

Fig. 7.11: Charlie Chaplin (out-toeing) gait

8

How to Interpret Examination Findings

(To arrive at a provisional and differential diagnosis)

+ Developmental dysplasia of the hip joint

+ Tom Smith arthritis

+ Perthes disease

+ Tuberculosis Hip

+ Spondyloarthropathy

+ Slipped capital femoral epiphysis

+ Old unreduced posterior dislocation of hip

+ Old Malunited intertrochanteric fracture

+ Non-union fracture neck of femur

+ Avascular necrosis

Common diseases affecting the hip, according to the age, are as under:

- **0–5 years** Developmental disorder of the hip (DDH), Tom Smith arthritis of hip joint, tuberculosis hip
- **5–15 years** Tuberculosis of hip joint, Perthes disease, SCFE (slipped capital femoral epiphysis), sequel of septic arthritis of the hip joint (Tom Smith arthritis), untreated or partially treated DDH, PPRP involving hip joint.
- **15–35 years** TB hip, ankylosing spondylitis/inflammatory arthritis affecting hip, untreated DDH, old unreduced dislocation of the hip, central fracture dislocation of the hip joint, PPRP of the hip joint, non-union fracture neck of femur, avascular necrosis (AVN) hip.
- **>35 years** TB hip, inflammatory arthritis (RA), old unreduced dislocation of the hip, malunited or neglected intertrochanteric fracture femur, non-union fracture neck of femur, avascular necrosis (AVN) hip, osteoarthritis primary or secondary.

Salient features which help in differentiating different affections of hip joint are described below.

DEVELOPMENTAL DYSPLASIA OF THE HIP JOINT

History: Sometimes it is diagnosed in a newborn infant by the attending paediatrician or staff nurse. If a child is few weeks of age, an intelligent mother may note an audible click during movements of hip joint (while changing diapers). When a child starts ambulation, parents notice limb length disparity, asymmetrical creases in upper thighs, and over a period of time—limp. Parents may also notice widened perineum in bilateral dislocations.

Examination: During examination, a clinician would appreciate asymmetrical gluteal and thigh folds, increased lumbar lordosis and widened perineum (in bilateral cases), and shortening of the affected limb. A child may have adducted attitude of the limb, femoral pulse/es are weakly palpable and there is proximal migration of the trochanter. A dislocated head may be palpable as a globular bony mass posteriorly. Abduction is restricted while internal rotation may be increased.

In a newborn or young infant, Barlow's and Ortolani's signs may be postitive. In later part of infancy, Galeazzi's sign will be positive and telescopy would be elicitable.

	Newborn and infants	*>2 years*
History	Limb length disparity, clicking sound while cleaning perineum, other congenital anomalies. Delayed walking	Shortened affected limb, abnormal gait, widened perineum (B/l case)
Gait	—	Unilateral—Trendelenburg, Bilateral—waddling
Inspection	Asymmetric gluteal and thigh folds, femoral shortening, widened perineum	Increased lumbar lordosis, shortening of affected limb, widened perineum (bilateral dislocation)
Palpation	Feeble femoral pulses, adduction attitude, head palpable out of acetabulum	Feeble femoral pulses (vascular sign of Narath positive), high ridding trochanter, head is out of acetabulum, adduction attitude
Movements	Abduction restricted	Abduction restricted, increased internal rotation
Measurements	Supratrochanteric shortening	Supratrochanteric shortening
Test	Barlow's and Ortoloni's sign positive	Galeazzi's sign positive, telescopy positive, Trendelenburg's sign positive
X-ray (Fig. 8.1)	Subluxated/dislocated hip	Dislocated hip

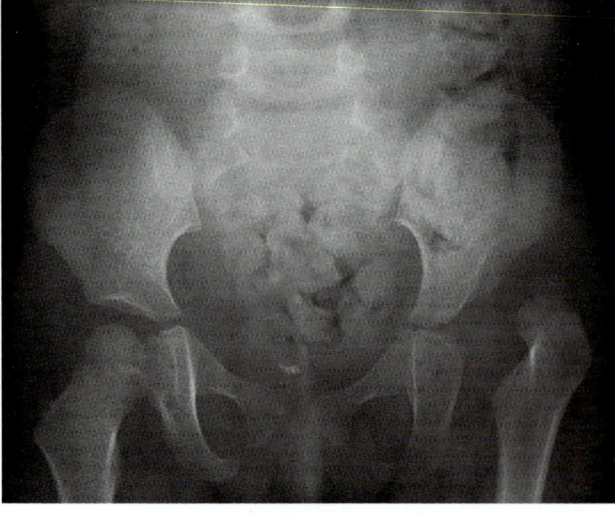

Fig. 8.1: Developmental dysplasia of the hip joint

TOM SMITH ARTHRITIS

Tom Smith arthritis (Fig. 8.2) of the hip or acute sepsis of the hip in infancy is unfortunately still not uncommon. Acute cases are real emergency because of vulnerability of mostly cartilaginous hip joints to the proteolytic enzymes, secreted by infective organisms and the body's defense cells which are trying to control infection.

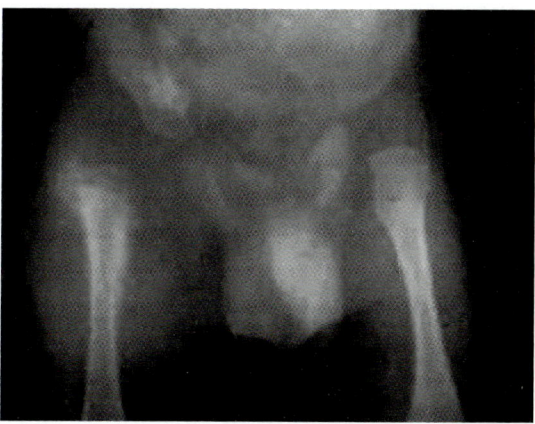

Fig. 8.2: Tom Smith arthritis

A clinician must be able to diagnose it to prevent disaster. A significant deviation from the usual picture of infection is lack of muscle spasm and presence of passive movements: In contrast to infection in older children, where spasm is pronounced and all attempts to move hip joint are resisted. The hapless victim of Tom Smith arthritis is suspected because of persistent crying, inability to move the limb, and refusal to take feeds. History of premature birth necessitating IV support and femoral vein puncture for investigations, gluteal injections, umbilical cord sepsis, may be present.

An examinee, however, would get a case of old Tom Smith arthritis. The child would have no pain and main complaint would be painless limp because of shortening and Trendelenburg gait. Tell-tale scars may be present on the hip. There would be obvious shortening and wasting of surrounding muscles. Trochanter would be high riding, and may be thick and irregular. Extent of destruction of upper end of the femur varies. In a case of gross destruction of head and neck, joint may be 'hypermobile', with increased range of movements in all directions. In a case of partial destruction, abduction and internal rotation are restricted to varying degrees. Trendelenburg test is positive and true supratrochanteric shortening would be seen.

	Acute case	Old case
History	History of premature birth, often necessitating IV support, umbilical cord sepsis, intramuscular injections in hip area, history of aspiration in the vicinity of hip joint or previous abscess drainage; persistent crying, inability to move the limb, and refusal to take feeds	Past history suggestive of infective arthritis hip in infancy or early childhood; painless limp because of shortening

Contd.

	Acute case	*Old case*
Gait	Inability to stand or walk	Trendelenburg gait, with short limb
Inspection	Limb may be in flexion, abduction, external rotation	Shortening, wasting of thigh/gluteal muscles, extragluteal crease, healed tell-tale scars
Palpation	Presence of passive movements due to lack of muscle spasm, in contrast to infection in older children where spasm is pronounced and all attempts to move hip joint are resistant	Femoral pulses absent/feeble (compared to other hip), trochanter is high may be thick and irregular
Movement	Normal passive movement	Gross destruction of head and neck—'hypermobile' joint; partial destruction—abduction and internal rotation restricted to varying degrees

PERTHES DISEASE

Also known as Legg-Calve-Perthes disease (Legg was from USA, Calve from France, and Perthes from Germany), other synonyms are—pseudocoxalgia, osteochondritis deformans, coxa juveniles, precoxalgia, coxa vara capitalis, coxa plana.

There is partial/almost complete avascular necrosis of the upper femoral epiphysis, without any apparent aetiology. It mostly follows a self-limiting course, with partial/complete recovery.

Commonly seen in 4–9 years old boys (male:Female—4:1), though can occur in the age group of 2–18 years. Prognosis is worse, if it occurs in later age (after 6 years)

The typical history is spontaneous and insidious onset of painless limp in an ambulatory child. In early stages, mild pain may also be present, which may sometimes be referred to the knee. Many years after the history of disease, the hip once again may become painful because of secondary degenerative arthritis.

The findings are relatively mild, compared to often alarming X-ray picture—mild wasting of thigh muscles, mild tenderness, some restriction of abduction and internal rotation, positive Trendelenburg sign, no fixed deformity, true supratrochanteric shortening of 1 cm or so.

Radiological findings will vary, according to the stage of the disease. Initially the X-ray may reveal only increase in medial joint space and smaller size of the upper femoral epiphyseal nucleus. A cystic area may be seen in the lateral part. Later, destruction and fragmentation of the ossification nucleus becomes apparent. There may also be flattening, decrease in height and lateral extrusion of the epiphysis. The metaphysis may show broadening and corresponding changes may also be seen in acetabulum. Eventually the reparative stage sets in with gradual revascularization and regain in density and size of the ossification nucleus. The flattening may not recover and lead to permanent changes (Fig. 8.3). Later in life—after 5th decade, secondary osteoarthritis sets in.

There are various classifications to indicate the severity of disease. Two common classifications used to grade Perthes disease are Catterall classification and Herring's lateral pillar classification. They are basically graded according to the amount of area and the collapse of the upper femoral epiphysis—higher the grade, more the area involved and bigger the collapse.

Herring's Lateral Pillar Classification (Table 8.1)

Table 8.1: Herring's lateral pillar classification		
Group A	Lateral pillar maintains full height without any density changes	
Group B	Maintains >50% height	
B/C border	Lateral pillar is narrowed (2–3 mm) or poorly ossified with approximately 50% height	
Group C	Less than 50% of lateral pillar height is maintained	

Catterall Classification (Table 8.2)

Table 8.2: Catterall classification		
Group 1	Involvement of the anterior epiphysis only	

Contd.

Table 8.2: Catterall classification (*Contd.*)

Group 2	Involvement of the anterior epiphysis with a central sequestrum	
Group 3	Only a small part of the epiphysis is not involved	
Group 4	Total head involvement	

Table 8.3: Perthes disease

History	Typically painless limp; mild pain in early stages referred to knee
Gait	Trendelenburg gait
Inspection	Wasting of thigh muscles, apparent shortening
Palpation	anterior hip tenderness
Movement	Decreased movements at hip joint in early course of disease (irritable hip); classical presentation—restriction of abduction and internal rotation
Measurement	Apparent shortening, mild true supratrochanteric shortening

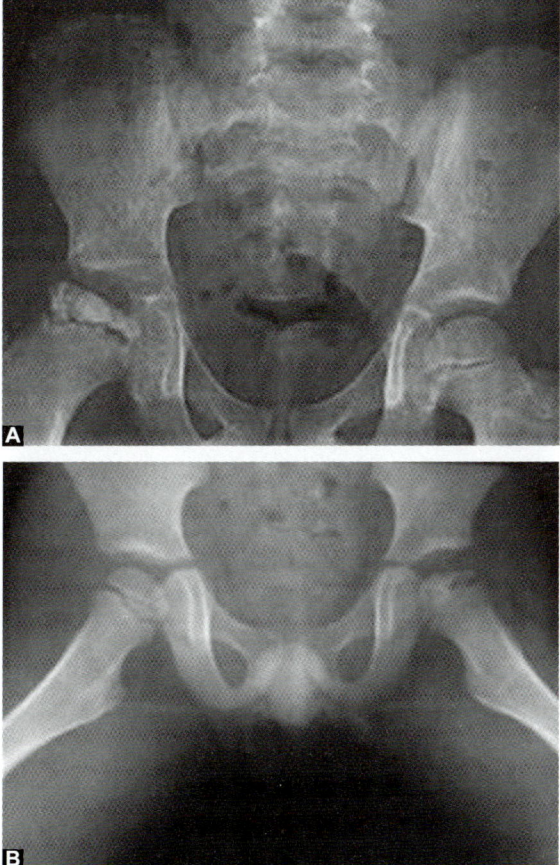

Fig. 8.3A and B: Perthes disease (Herring's group C, Catterall group 4): (A) AP view; (B) Frog leg lateral view

TUBERCULOSIS HIP

Tuberculosis of the hip joint is a common type of osteoarticular tuberculosis, with far reaching consequences on ambulation and activities of daily life. Hip joint tuberculosis occurs more commonly in young adolescents, but can occur in any age group. The usual clinical picture insidious onset of hip pain, painful limp, associated with constitutional symptoms—weight loss, loss of appetite, low grade fever in evening and malaise. A history of contact with a tubercular patient in family, or neighbourhood is common. There may also be history of having taken antitubercular treatment for tuberculosis elsewhere in the body. History of night cries, i.e. waking up from sleep with a painful cry is typically seen in young patients. It is because of inflamed articular surfaces coming in contact, due to release of muscle spasm during sleep. History of discharging sinus or a swelling (cold abscess) in the vicinity of the joint may be there.

Classically tuberculosis of the hip joint has been described to have four stages:

1. **Stage of synovitis:** Hip joint is in an attitude of flexion, abduction and external rotation. Patients rarely report in this stage. Diagnosis may also be missed, even if they report at this stage.

2. **Stage of early arthritis:** The joint is fixed in flexion, adduction and internal rotation of varying degree.
3. **Stage of advanced arthritis:** There is severe flexion, adduction and internal rotation deformity.
4. **Stage of wandering acetabulum:** Destruction of the acetabulum in the superolateral part leads to subluxation/dislocation of the destroyed head.

However, in the present day orthopaedic practice, the stages and their associated deformities are often altered by treatment taken (mostly incomplete ATT), traction and manipulation.

The hallmark of disease remains constitutional symptoms and muscle wasting. It must be re-emphasised that the muscle wasting is more than expected, i.e. it is quite prolonged and obvious.

Examination

If the patient is able to ambulate, the gait is usually antalgic and Trendelenburg component may also be present. Ambulation may only be possible with some support. A physical examination may reveal the extent of abduction/adduction deformity, hip tenderness and global restriction of movements. Adductor and lower abdominal muscle spasm is often obvious and there is gross resistance on attempted movements of hip joint. Wasting of the gluteal and thigh muscles is obvious and pronounced. Shortening, both apparent and true, would be present. In many late stages, dislocated and destroyed head may be palpable in the gluteal region. In this stage, the femoral pulses may be feeble.

X-ray

Destruction of the joint is the hallmark. There is variable degree of destruction of head of femur and acetabulum, joint space is reduced, articular and periarticular rarefaction is obvious. In late stages, wandering acetabulum, i.e. destruction of superolateral part of acetabulum with subluxation of head of femur, is present. Soft tissue swelling may be seen. For detailed description of radiological findings, please refer to Chapter on X-ray Findings.

SPONDYLOARTHROPATHY/INFLAMMATORY ARTHRITIS

The possible common clinical diagnoses in case of non-infective inflammatory arthritis of the hip joint are rheumatoid arthritis and ankylosing spondylitis. The rare causes would include SLE, crystal arthropathy (mainly gout), psoriatic arthropathy. The first two are more relevant and warrant detailed description. The two in fact belong to two distinct groups of inflammatory arthritis—seropositive and seronegative spondylo-arthropathies (since both of them have involvement of spine and peripheral joints). Spine involvement is more pronounced in ankylosing arthritis while peripheral joints are more severely affected in rheumatoid arthritis. However, in advanced stages, spine and other joints are equally damaged. The two groups are differentiated by the presence of RA factor and ANA bodies in the seropositive group, whereas these two are absent in the seronegative group. In the seronegative group, there is presence of HLA B27.

Rheumatoid Arthritis (Fig. 8.4)

This chronic inflammatory systemic disease is more common in middle-aged females. Involvement of joints other than hip, particularly small joints of the hand and wrist, is obvious and common. Hip joints are affected in advanced cases. Simultaneous involvement of contralateral hip and the knee joints may make the patient bedridden. The affected hip joint has commonly flexion, adduction and internal rotation deformity. The joint is tender, there is supratrochanteric shortening and all movements are painful. The X-ray reveals a grossly destroyed joint with varying degrees of damage to the head as well as acetabulum. Destruction of the acetabular floor may lead to protusio acetabuli (Fig. 8.4). Reduced bone density is obvious and soft tissue swelling may be appreciated. Laboratory investigations would reveal raised ESR, strongly positive RA factor, presence of anti-CCP and ANA, and raised CRP. Cervical spine is more commonly involved than other regions of the spine.

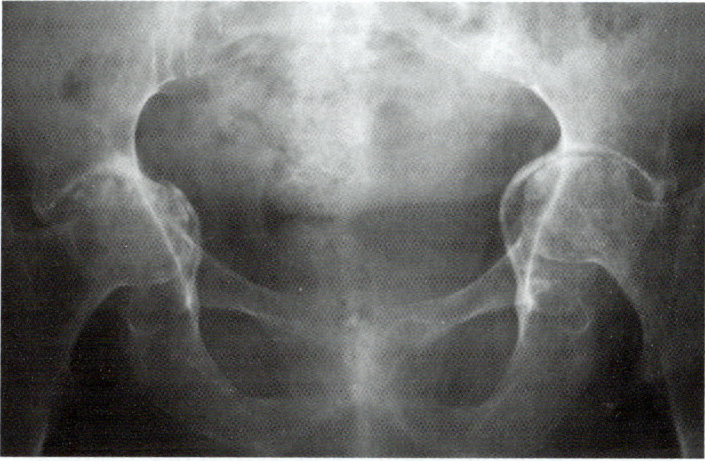

Fig. 8.4: Rheumatoid arthritis

Ankylosing Spondylitis (Fig. 8.5)

Ankylosing spondylitis (AS) is the commonest and most important type of seronegative spondyloarthropathies. Three other entities in group include psoriatic arthritis, reactive arthritis (Reiter's syndrome) and enteropathic arthropathy.

Ankylosing spondylitis occurs mostly in males in 3rd or 4th decade. The male to female ratio is almost 6:1. The disease almost always starts with the involvement of the spine and sacroiliac joints are invariably almost involved. The dorsolumbar regions of the spine are affected while the cervical spine is spared which is in contrast to rheumatoid arthritis where cervical spine is the region of spine affected. Hip and other large joints are involved in later part of the disease. The patient may become bedridden once spine, hip and knee are involved.

Deformities of the hip joint are variable, depending upon the posture and the built, treatment in the form of traction etc. Combination of deformities is seen and the two hips may have many different deformities. In the initial stage of hip involvement, there is tenderness and painful restriction of all movements; while in later stages painless absence of movement i.e. bony ankylosis of the hip joint is the hallmark of the disease. Supra trochanteric shortening is always present, once the hip joint is involved.

Investigations may reveal raised ESR, increased CRP and presence of HLA B27 antigen. X-rays usually show para spinal calcification, leading ultimately to bamboo spine, obliteration (later absence) of sacroiliac joint space and ankylosis of hip joints (Fig. 8.5). The spine, sacroiliac joint and hip joint may look like a single bone, which leads to ankylosed spine and stiff hip gait in these patients.

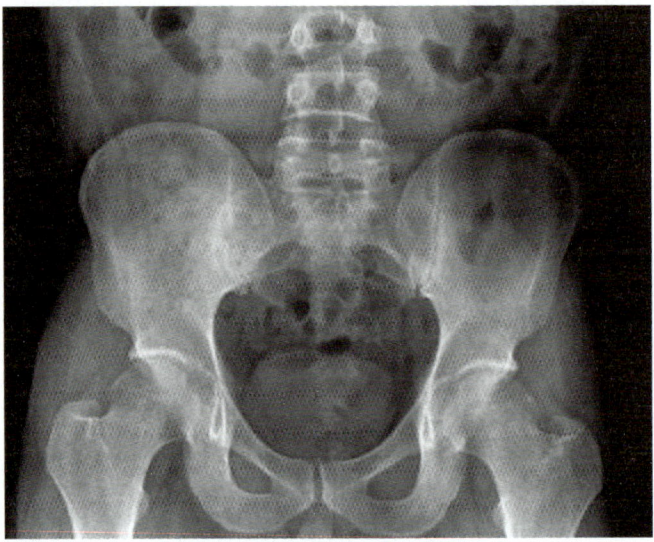

Fig. 8.5: Ankylosing spondylitis

SLIPPED CAPITAL FEMORAL EPIPHYSIS

It is a chronic, gradual slip of upper femoral epiphysis in a posteroinferior direction. The exact aetiology is not known, history of some form of trauma may be there. It is a disease of the adolescence more common in males. Typical body type described is overweight and features of hypogonadism may be present. The disease is very often bilateral—up to 60% of cases.

Presenting complaints are gradual onset of pain on anterior aspect of hip or the knee. Painful limp may appear and a gradually increasing *external rotation deformity of the lower limb* may become obvious. Mild flexion deformity may be there. Abduction and internal rotation are restricted. Supratrochanteric shortening and increase in length of the hypotenuse of Bryant's triangle, i.e. distance between anterior superior iliac spine and tip of greater trochanter, are obvious.

X-rays (Fig. 8.6), particularly lateral views, reveal the slip. Treatment includes, either fixation *in situ*, or gentle open reduction and fixation, or corrective femoral osteotomy, depending upon the stage and severity of the disease.

OLD UNREDUCED POSTERIOR DISLOCATION OF HIP (Fig. 8.7)

Unfortunately neglected cases of the posterior dislocation of the hip are still encountered in our country. Following a severe trauma to the hip, the posterior dislocation was either managed inadequately or inappropriately. Patient is usually a young adult, who is able to ambulate after a few weeks of rest. The hip which was initially painful in the

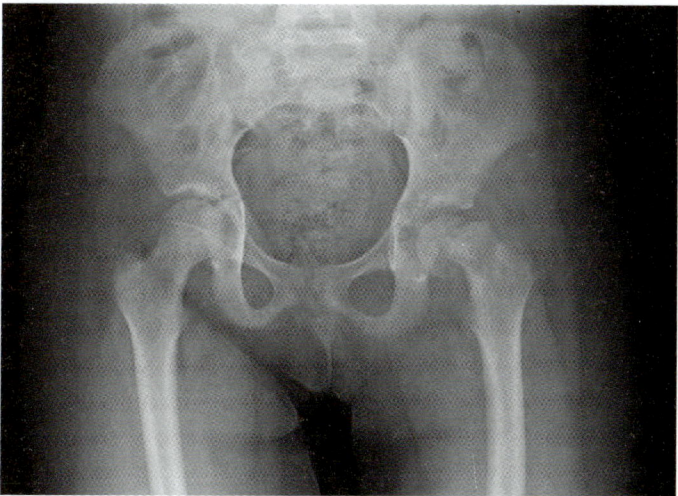

Fig. 8.6: Slipped capital femoral epiphysis

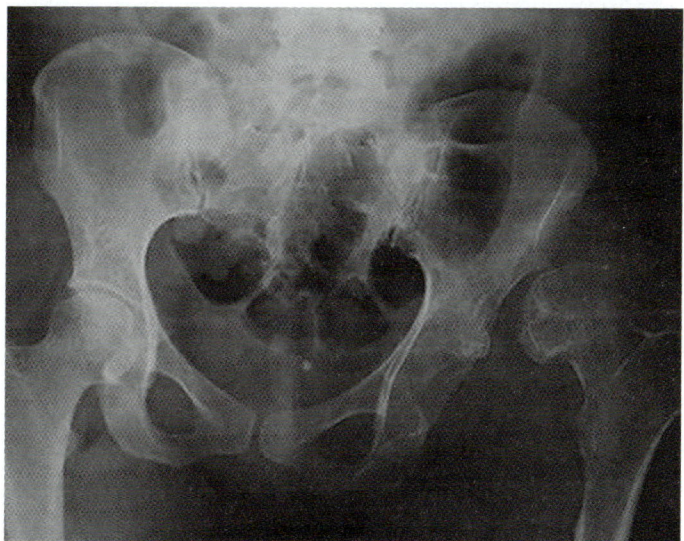

Fig. 8.7: Old unreduced posterior dislocation of hip

beginning of ambulation, gradually becomes painless. The pain would re-appear in advance age because of secondary osteoarthritis. The patient is usually able to walk without support. The patient reports for treatment for shortening, abnormal gait and later appearance of pain.

The patient has Trendelenburg and short limb gait. Shortening of the limb, undue protuberance of the gluteal region and exaggerated lumbar lordosis are apparent. Wasting of thigh muscles may be seen. On palpation, deep tenderness may be present. Trochanter is proximally migrated, sometimes to the extent of reversal of Bryant's triangle. Vascular sign of Narath is present, i.e. femoral pulses are palpable feebly in comparison to normal side. An abnormal globular, bony mass, which conforms to the shape of head of femur, is palpable in the gluteal region, and it moves with the movement of shaft of femur. This particular finding and presence of telescoping clinches the diagnosis. A fixed flexion deformity is likely; while abduction–adduction, internal–external rotation are pain free and are either almost complete or may even be increased in range. True supratrochanteric shortening of 3 or more centimetres is present.

OLD MALUNITED INTERTROCHANTERIC FRACTURE (Fig. 8.8)

Patient is usually an elderly one, who sustained the hip injury after a trivial trauma, e.g. slipping in the washroom. Uncommonly, younger patients have this injury following a major accident. Malunion follows an inadequate or inappropriate treatment. These fractures unite, even in absence of treatment and non-union is very rare. In a malunited intertrochanteric fracture, patient is able to walk with minimal assistance like a walking stick. In younger patients who are able to stand on one leg, Trendelenburg test may be positive. The limb is in external rotation. Patients walk with a short limb and Trendelenburg gait. On examination, the limb is in external rotation, with patella and foot pointing outwards, shortening is obvious and wasting of thigh muscles is there. On palpation, there is hardly any tenderness. The major guiding finding is broad, roughened and thickened trochanter. Proximal migration of greater trochanter (because of coxa vara) is likely. Consequently, the base of the Bryant's triangle is smaller and leads to supratrochanteric shortening. Active SLR is possible. Due to coxa vara, abduction is restricted, and due to fixed external rotation deformity, internal rotation is absent. Other movements are almost complete and painless. True supratrochanteric shortening of 2–3 cm and wasting of the thigh circumference is present.

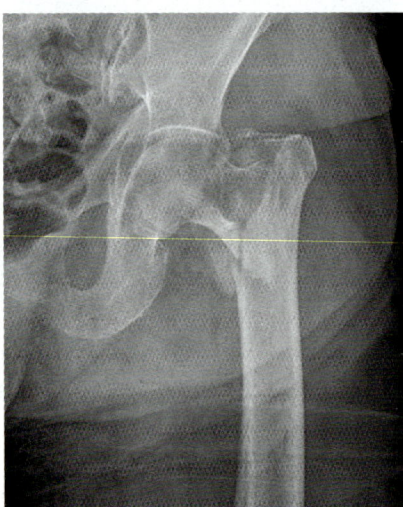

Fig. 8.8: Old malunited intertrochanteric fracture

NON-UNION FRACTURE NECK OF FEMUR (Fig. 8.9)

Patient is either an elderly, who sustained neck of femur fracture following a minor trauma, or a young person involved in a major traumatic event. Either no expert treatment has been taken, or the treatment has failed. Patient of established non-union of the neck of femur needs assistance for ambulation. A walking stick or crutches may

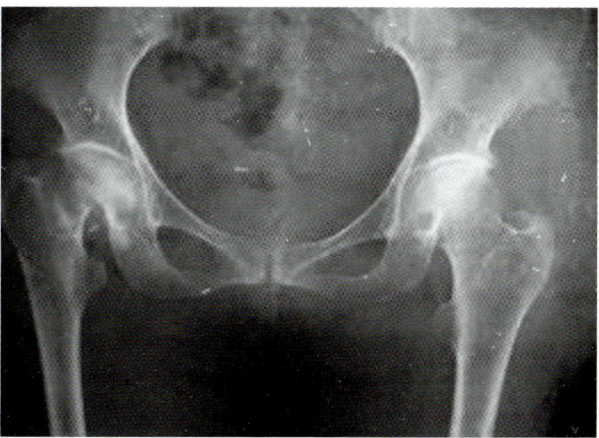

Fig. 8.9: Non-union fracture neck of femur

be required. Patient is not able to perform Trendelenburg test. On inspection, the limb is obviously short and is in an attitude of external rotation. The degree of external rotation of the limb is less than that seen in a case of malunited intertrochanteric fracture. On palpation, there is no fixed deformity and trochanter is normal in shape and texture. There is likely to be supratrochanteric shortening of about 2 cm (less than that seen in cases of malunited intertrochanteric fracture). The patient is not able to perform active straight leg raising. There is hardly any restriction of hip movements—*rather the movements are increased in range*, since these are occurring at the fracture site. The confirmatory finding would be telescoping, which is occurring at the fracture site. There is true supratrochanteric shortening and some amount of wasting of thigh muscles.

AVASCULAR NECROSIS (Fig. 8.10)

Avascular necrosis of the head of the femur is probably the commonest reason to perform total hip replacement in middle age. AVN of the hip can result from various causes—steroid intake, alcohol abuse, hemoglobinopathies and following trauma. In a

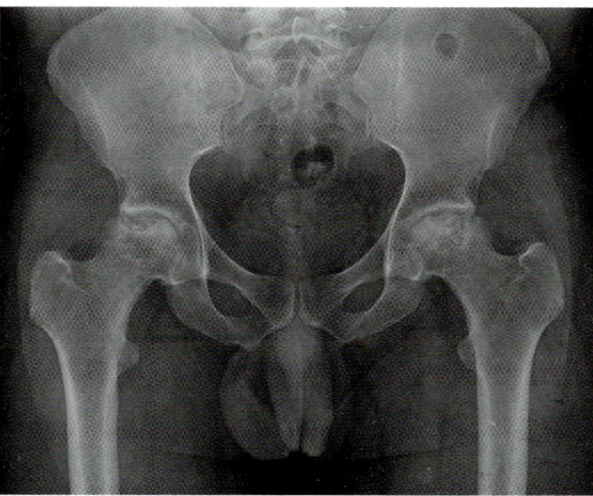

Fig. 8.10: Avascular necrosis

few cases, inspite of extensive history and investigations, the reason remains unknown, i.e. idiopathic. Except for post-traumatic cases, other patients may develop bilateral disease.

In suspected cases of AVN of the hip, history of steroid intake and alcohol abuse must be inquired. Other relevant history to be elicited would be to rule out hemoglobinopathies like sickle cell disease, and enzyme disorders like Gaucher's disease. There may be old history of significant trauma, and surgery in post-traumatic cases. Patient is typically young or middle aged and presents with pain, which is spontaneous (except post-traumatic) and insidious in onset. Patient has an antalgic Trendelenburg gait. In bilateral cases, there may be waddling gait. As the disease progresses, patient may require the use of a cane or stick to ambulate.

On examination, patient has anterior hip tenderness and mild wasting of the thigh. Mild flexion deformity is common. Fixed deformity in the coronal plane may not be there. If such a deformity is present, it is usually adduction deformity and uncommonly abduction deformity. Rotational deformities are also mild in extent. There is painful restriction of movements, though not as gross as in cases of inflammatory arthritis. True supratrochanteric shortening of 1.5–2 cm is present. A significant and often diagnostic finding on checking movements is the presence of axes deviation or so-called sectoral sign. This finding is positive, if on attempted on passive flexion of the hip, hip cannot be flexed beyond 80/90° unless it is moved in a slightly deviated access of mild abduction and external rotation. It means that a flexion beyond 90° is not possible in neutral axes, but is present in deviated axes of mild abduction and external rotation. This finding is explained on the fact that on attempted passive flexion of the hip joint, when the diseased and deformed area of the femoral head comes in contact with acetabulum and prevents flexion beyond 90°; and when hip is slightly abducted and externally rotated, a comparatively normal area of the femoral head comes in contact with the acetabulum and allows further flexion. The other hip must be examined to look for early signs of AVN.

How to Interpret
Hip Radiographs

<table>
<tr><td>✦ Importance of X-ray</td><td>✦ Acetabulum</td></tr>
<tr><td>✦ Different radiographic views</td><td>✦ Head-neck characteristics including offset</td></tr>
<tr><td>✦ Interpretation of soft tissue</td><td>✦ Radiographic findings in different hip diseases</td></tr>
<tr><td>✦ Interpretation of bony elements</td><td></td></tr>
</table>

IMPORTANCE OF X-RAY

Plain radiograph is the basic and essential investigation in any orthopaedic patient. It will not be an exaggeration to state that significance of a plain radiograph for an orthopaedic surgeon is same as that of a haemogram for a practicing general physician. An orthopaedic surgeon must think of a plain radiograph before any other investigation, in every patient of orthopaedic disease.

Radiology has evolved tremendously over past a few years and several types of radiological investigations are now available—like CT, MRI, bone scan, PET scan, etc. However, a plain radiograph can provide certain information, which may not be available with other radiological methods—for example, bird's eye view of the pelvis, architectural composition (bony trabeculae) of the part under view, obvious side/site of pathology in a quick glance, etc. The utility of plain radiograph, as a cost-effective and easily available investigations, is unparalleled.

DIFFERENT RADIOGRAPHIC VIEWS

A standard anteroposterior view of the pelvis with both hips, and a lateral view (cross-table lateral/frog leg) are the bare minimum. Special views can be done whenever indicated.

AP Radiograph of the Pelvis

The anteroposterior pelvic radiograph is taken with the patient lying supine on the X-ray table, and both lower extremities in 15° of internal rotation. When the hip is in 15°of internal rotation, it neutralizes the anatomical anteversion of the neck of the femur. In this position, the neck comes to lie parallel to the X-ray cassette and the complete profile of the neck can be seen. In the normally present 10° of external rotation attitude of the limb, complete profile of the neck of the femur cannot be seen. Even after the X-ray has been taken, one can find out whether the hip was in internal rotation or not, when it was X-rayed. The profile of the lesser trochanter, visible in the available X-ray, indicates this. If the hip is in internal rotation, the lesser trochanter which is anatomically postromedial becomes more posterior and is hardly visible on the X-ray. In comparison, if the limb was in external rotation, when the hip was X-rayed, the lesser trochanter, from its postromedial position becomes medial, and is prominently visible on the X-ray (Fig. 9.1A and B). This has a practical significance in cases of suspected fracture neck femur—the level of the fracture and the remaining neck length will be important for type of surgery as well as to predict the prognosis (Fig. 9.1C and D).

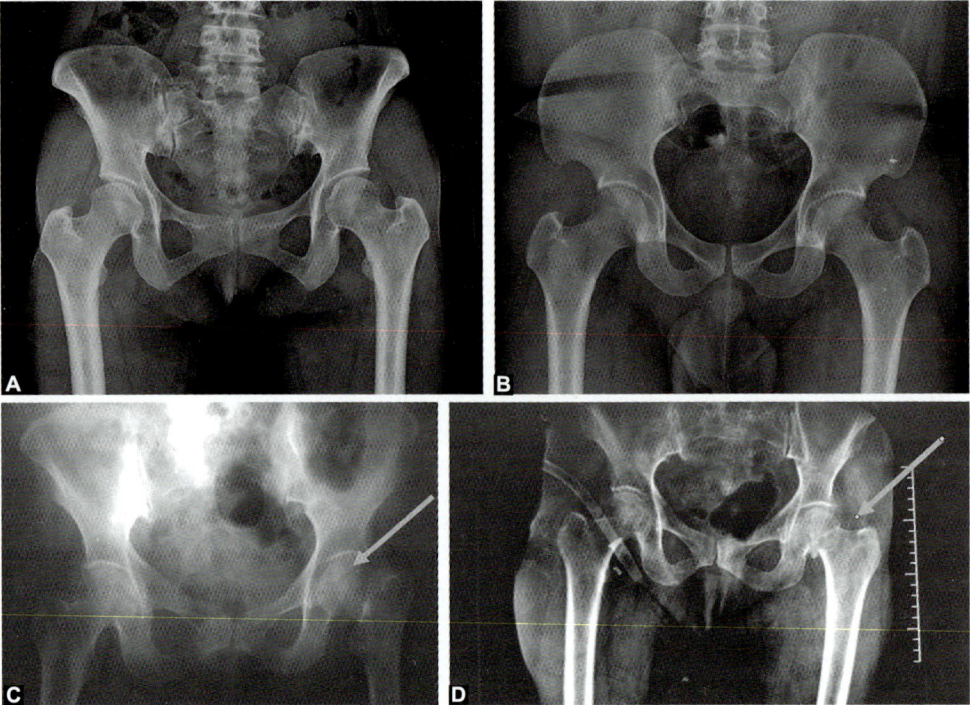

Fig. 9.1A to D: AP view of normal pelvis with both hips: (A) Lower extremities in normal 10° external rotation; (B) Lower extremities in 15° external rotation; (C) Fracture neck femur—left side, limb in external rotation; (D) Fracture neck femur—left side, limb in internal rotation compare the length of the neck femur and position of lesser trochanter.

The X-ray tube-to-film distance should be 120 cm, with the tube oriented perpendicular to the table. The focus of the beam should be at just above pubic symphysis centre (Fig. 9.2).

In an AP radiograph of a normal hip, following observations can be made (Fig. 9.3):
- Symphysis pubis—less than 5 mm in width
- Sacroiliac joint 2–4 mm in width
- Pelvic ring should have no disruption
- Obturator ring should have no disruption
- Sacral foraminal lines should be clearly visible

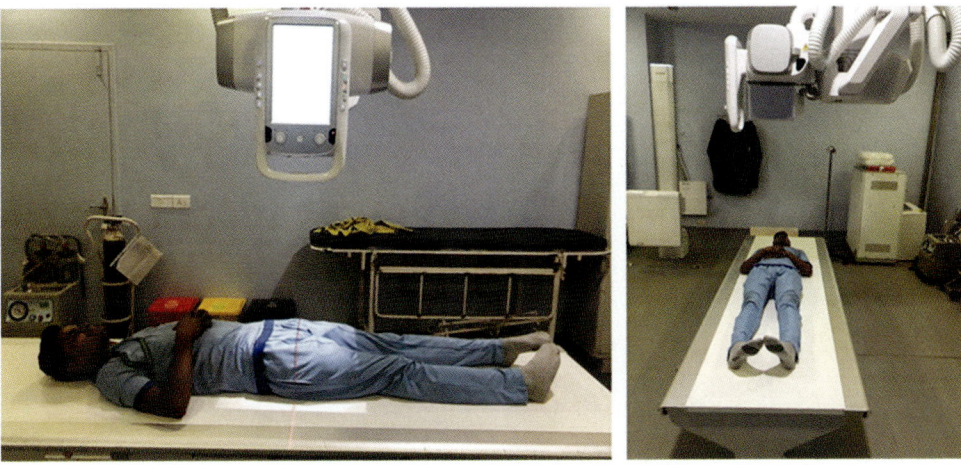

Fig. 9.2: Position of patient while performing AP view of pelvis

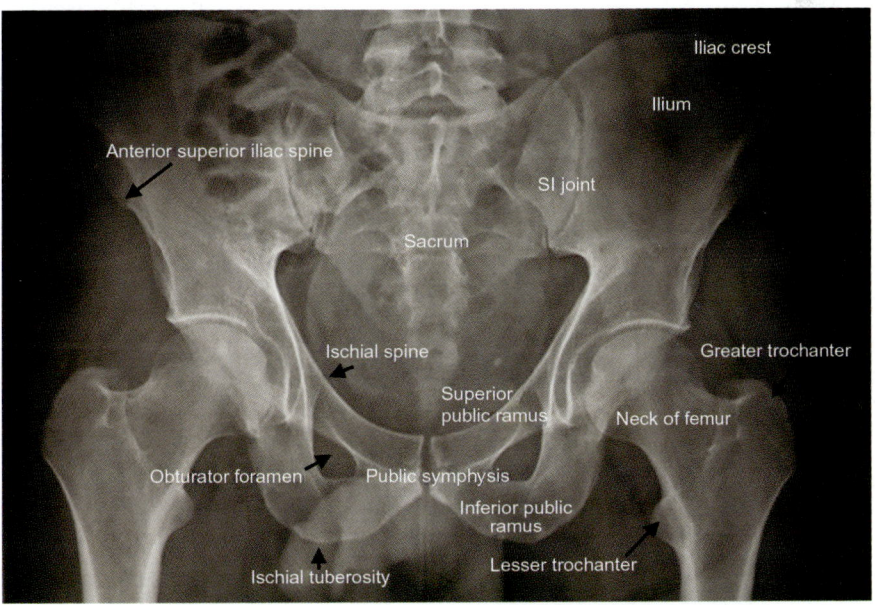

Fig. 9.3: AP view of pelvis showing various landmarks

Cross-Table Lateral View (Fig. 9.4)

The cross-table lateral radiograph is taken with the patient lying supine on the X-ray table. The contralateral hip and knee are flexed beyond 80°, and the affected limb is straight and 15° internally rotated. The X-ray beam should be parallel to the table and oriented at a 45° angle to the affected limb, centered at femoral head. The cassette is kept along the ilium at an angle of 45°.

This view has the advantage that the limb and the hip joint need not be moved and so this view can be done easily in a painful hip joint. However, both hips cannot be X-rayed at the same time.

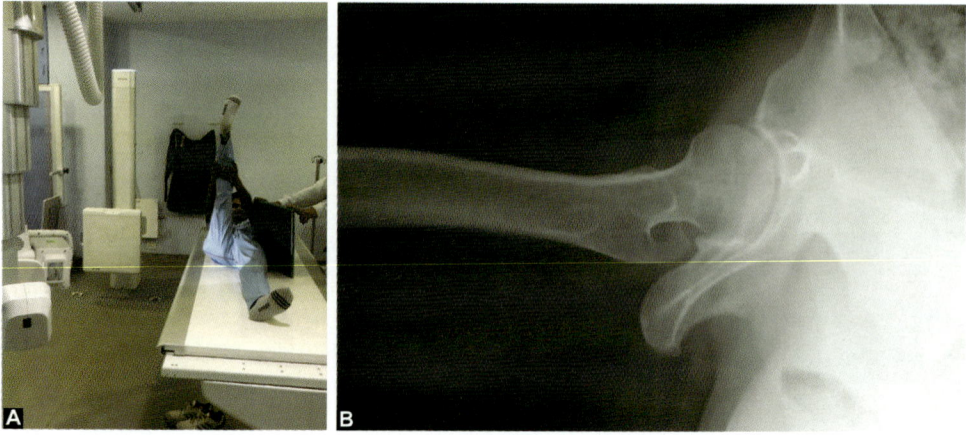

Fig. 9.4A and B: Cross-table lateral view: (A) Position of patient; (B) X-ray of cross-table lateral view.

Frog-Leg Lateral View

In place of cross-table lateral view, the lateral profile of the hip joint can be seen by another method, called frog-leg lateral view (Fig. 9.5).

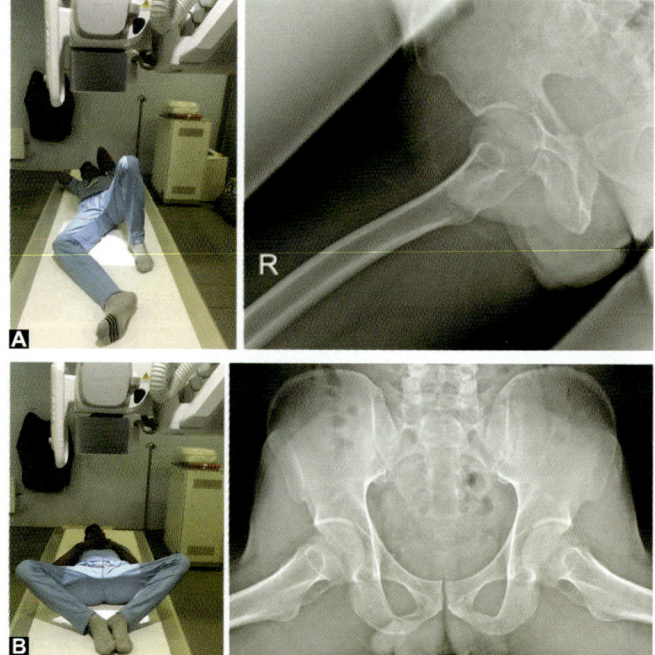

Fig. 9.5A and B: Frog-leg lateral view: (A) One hip; (B) Both hips

To take a frog-leg lateral radiograph of the hip, the patient should be positioned supine on the X-ray table. The affected limb is positioned in a way that the knee is flexed about 40°, and the hip is flexed, abducted 45° and externally rotated, so that the heel of the limb comes to touch the medial aspect of the opposite knee. This resembles a figure of four position. The cassette is kept behind the hip and the beam is directed at 90° to centre of femoral head. Painless range of motion in the hip is a pre-requisite for this view. By placing the other hip in a similar degree of flexion, abduction and external rotation, and centering the X-ray beam over the pubic symphysis, both the hips can be viewed in lateral profile, simultaneously.

The characteristics of the above views have been summarized in Table 9.1.

Table 9.1: Various views of hip radiographs			
View	*Method*	*Illustration*	*Characteristics*
1. Anteroposterior view	✖ Patient supine; both feet in 15° of internal rotation ✖ X-ray tube at 120 cm ✖ Focus of beam just above pubic symphysis		✖ Symphysis pubis <5 mm ✖ Sacroiliac joint 2–4 mm ✖ Pelvic ring and obturator without disruption
2. Cross-table lateral view	✖ Patient supine; contralateral hip and knee flexed beyond 80°; affected limb internally rotated by 15° ✖ Beam centred at femoral head, oriented at 45° to affected limb ✖ Cassette kept along ilium at 45°		✖ Advantage: Limb and hip joint need not be moved ✖ Easily done in painful hip joint ✖ Disadvantage: Both hips cannot be X-rayed simultaneously
3. Frog-leg lateral view	✖ Patient supine; feet together, thighs maximally abducted and externally rotated ✖ X-ray tube at 40 inches (102 cm) ✖ Beam directed just above pubic symphysis		✖ Prerequisite painless range of motion in hip ✖ Both hip joints can be X-rayed on same film

Special Views

Other views, which can be taken in a case of hip joint disease, are as follows:

1. Iliac oblique
2. Obturator oblique
3. Pelvic inlet
4. Pelvic outlet

These special views are required in specific cases, depending on the particular information sought. Table 9.2 provides the details of the special views and the information they provide.

Table 9.2: Special views of hip radiograph

View	Method	Illustration	Characteristics
1. Anterior (obturator) oblique view	✗ Patient supine; affected side rotated anteriorly 45° ✗ Beam directed vertically towards affected hip		✗ Shows iliopectineal line (anterior column) of pelvis and posterior wall
2. Posterior (iliac) oblique view	✗ Patient supine; uninvolved side rotated anteriorly 45° ✗ Beam directed vertically towards the affected hip		✗ Shows ilioischial line (posterior column) and anterior wall
3. Pelvic inlet view	✗ Patient supine ✗ Tube angled 30–35° caudal ✗ Beam directed at centre of pelvis		✗ Sacral promontory, iliopectineal line (anterior column), ischial spine, pubic symphysis visualized
4. Pelvic outlet (Ferguson) view	✗ Patient supine ✗ Tube angled 30–35° cephalad ✗ Beam directed at center of pelvis		✗ Sacroiliac joints, pubic rami, posterior acetabular rim visualized

READING X-RAY—INTERPRETATION OF SOFT TISSUE

In a good radiograph, it is possible to get an idea of the soft tissue status, around the hip. One should make a note of any abnormal soft tissue shadow in the pelvic area, which may indicate a soft tissue tumour or an abscess. Look specifically for details of the iliopsoas muscle outline—it may be more prominent on one side in a case of cold abscess. Look for calcification of obturator membrane, which may indicate fluorosis, not an uncommon finding in patients particularly in the northern belt of India (Punjab, Haryana, and Rajasthan). Sometimes, the calcification of obturator membrane may be seen in patients of ankylosing spondylitis (Fig. 9.6).

A few fat planes have been described in AP radiograph of pelvis. These can be appreciated only in good quality X-rays.

Some consistent fat planes, occurring in radiographs of pelvis with both hips, are given in Table 9.3.

Table 9.3: Interpretation of soft tissues on pelvis X-rays		
Name of the fat plane	Description	Significance
1. Gluteal fat stripe	Straight line parallel to superior aspect of femoral neck; represents normal fat between gluteus minimus tendon and hip joint capsule	In hip joint effusion, line bulges superiorly
2. Iliopsoas fat stripe	Lucent line, just inferior to iliopsoas tendon insertion	Displaced in iliopsoas tendon avulsion/cold abcess
3. Obturator fat stripe	Lucent line parallel to iliopectineal line; represents fat in the vicinity of obturator internus muscle	Displaced in presence of fracture haematoma or a mass

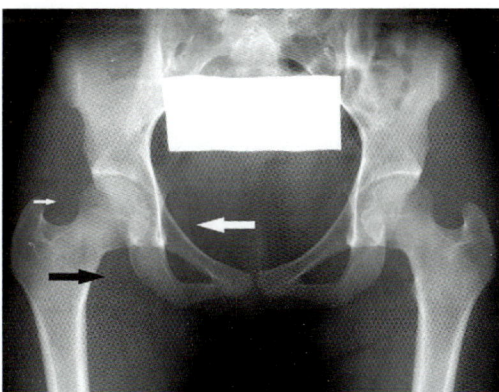

Fig. 9.6: AP view of pelvis showing soft tissue shadows. {The gluteus minimus fat stripe (small white arrow), obturator internus fat stripe (large white arrow), and iliopsoas fat stripe (black arrow).}

READING AN X-RAY—INTERPRETATION OF BONY ELEMENTS (Fig. 9.7)

A quick general assessment of the bony pelvis is done; and any obvious pathology is noted, e.g. multiple lytic areas of hyperparathyroidism (with a pathological fracture neck femur), any evident primary or secondary tumour, features of metabolic bone disease like osteomalacia (Looser's line), etc.

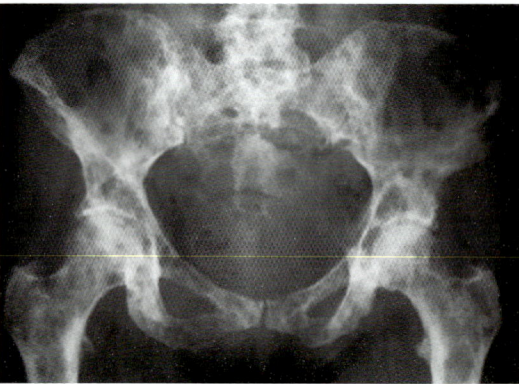

Fig. 9.7: X-ray of pelvis showing wide-spread metastasis.

Attention is then focused, specifically to the bones of the hip joint, i.e. acetabulum, and head and neck of femur. To interpret findings in these two, a few radiographic lines have been described:

1. **Iliopectineal line (ileopubic line):** This line extends from the medial border of the iliac wing, along the superior border of the superior pubic ramus and ends at the pubic symphysis. It defines the anterior column of the hemipelvis on that side. The two iliopectineal lines of the two sides together form the margins of the pelvic brim. This line is disrupted in cases of fractures of the anterior column of pelvis (Fig. 9.8).

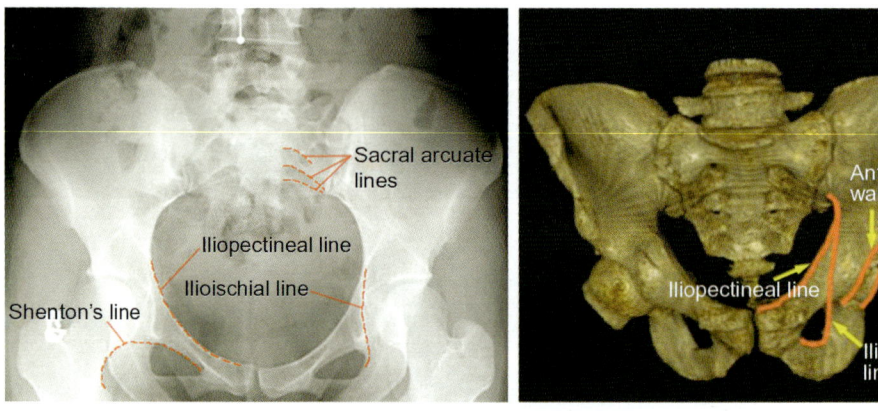

Fig. 9.8: Various radiographic line in AP view of pelvis

2. **Ilioischial line:** This line begins at the medial border of the iliac wing and extends along the medial border of the ischium to end at the ischial tuberosity. This defines the posterior column of the pelvis. It is broken in the fractures of the posterior column (Fig. 9.8).
3. **Shenton line:** It is a smooth curvilinear line, connecting the medial aspect of the femoral neck with the under surface of the superior pubic ramus. It is disrupted in destruction of head and neck of femur, which could be because of several causes like infection, AVN, (Fig. 9.8) etc.
4. **Paediatrics hip lines** (Fig. 9.9)
   a. *Hilgenreiner's line:* A horizontal line connecting centres of triradiate cartilage of the two sides.

b. *Perkin's line:* Vertical line along lateral edge of triradiate cartilage.
These lines divide the hip joint space into four quadrants (superolateral, inferolateral, superomedial and inferomedial quadrants). The upper femoral epiphysis should be seen in the inferomedial quadrant: It should be normally located below Hilgenreiner's line, and medial to Perkin line. If it is not , the hip is subluxated or dislocated.

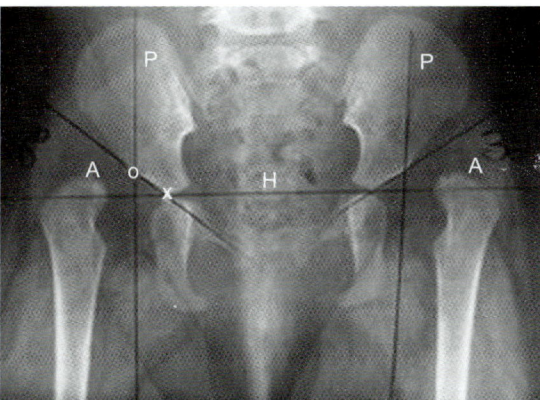

H - Hillgenreiner's line
P - Perkin's line
x - Triadiate cartilage
o - Lateral border of
    acetabulum

Fig. 9.9: Radiographic line in paediatric hip

c. *Line of Klein:* The line of Klein describes a line along the superior edge of the neck of femur. It is useful in detecting early slipped capital femoral epiphysis (SCFE) in adolescents. The line should normally intersect the lateral part of the superior femoral epiphysis. The line fails to intersect the epiphysis, if the epiphysis has slipped (Fig. 9.10). This finding is called Trethowan's sign.

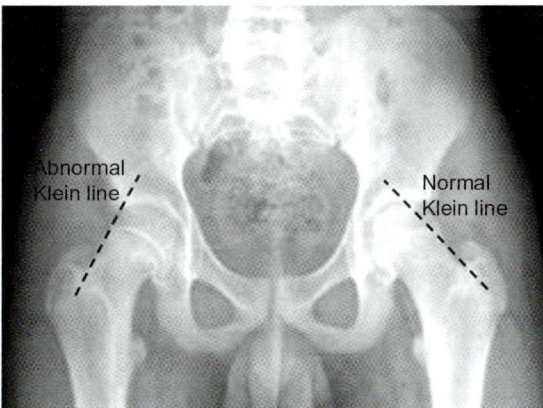

Fig. 9.10: Early SCFE in right hip

ACETABULUM

There are several points, which are to be observed, when commenting about status of the acetabulum in a plain radiograph of the pelvis with both the hips.

A few points concern with general features like shape, outline and regularity. A few specialized characteristics have to be specially derived or calculated like inclination, depth, version, etc. The different headings under which the acetabulum can be assessed radiographically are:

1. General configuration
2. Tear drop
3. Sourcil
4. Acetabular index
5. Acetabular depth
6. Acetabular version
7. Congruency

General Configuration

Make a note of the general outline of the acetabulum—whether it is regular or broken. A common pattern of disturbed outline of the acetabulum is superior migration of acetabulum. It is infact destruction of the superolateral part of the acetabulum because of a disease like tuberculosis/infection. The weakened and soft superolateral part of acetabulum is indented by the pressure of the femoral head, during weight bearing. The femoral head seems to move superiorly through the destroyed bone. The lateral part of the acetabulum appears deeper than the rest of the acetabulum and is named as superior migration of acetabulum. In advance cases, it is called 'wandering' acetabulum.

Tear Drop

It is a radiographic finding and named so, because it resembles a falling tear. It is located along the medial aspect of acetabular floor. The appearance of the tear is because of the typical configuration of the ischium bone contributing to the floor of the acetabulum. A small part of the tear is contributed by superior pubic ramus. The distance between the medial border of the femoral head and the lateral margin of tear drop is equal on the two sides. This distance will be disturbed in hip joint effusion, dysplasia of the hip, etc. The tear drop may be misshapen in destructive diseases of the hip joint (Fig. 9.11).

Sourcil

Sourcil is a French word, which literally means 'eyebrow', the sclerosed outline of the lateral border of the acetabulum resembles an eyebrow, and hence the name. The sourcil would be disturbed in cases of any hip arthritis which destroys acetabulum.

Acetabular Index

The inclination of the acetabular wall is crucial to determine the stability of the hip joint—if the acetabulum is more vertical, the hip is unstable. The exact inclination of acetabulum is estimated by calculating acetabulum index:
• A line is drawn connecting the lateral margin of acetabular roof (Sourcil) and the inferior aspect of the tear drop.

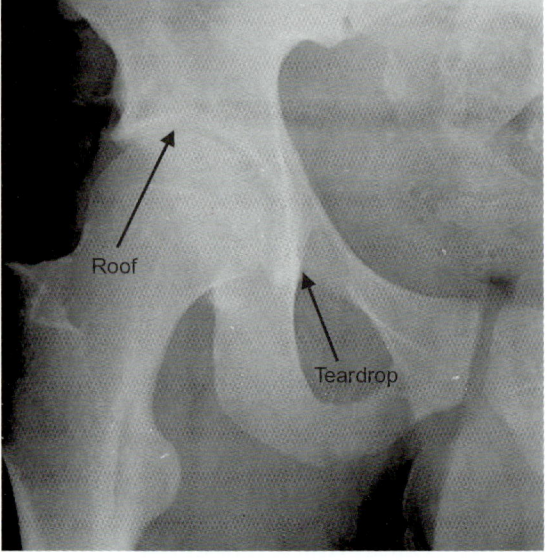

Roof

Teardrop

Fig. 9.11: Tear drop

- Another line is drawn horizontally, connecting the inferior aspects of the two tear drops.
- Angle between these lines are called acetabular index, normally it is less than 30°.

Acetabular Depth

The depth of the acetabulum is measured in relation to the ileoischial line. Normally the acetabular depth is such that the outline of the femur head lies just lateral to ileoischial line. If the acetabular depth is such that the outline of the head of femur goes medial to the ileoischial line, the depth is increased—such an acetabulum is called protusio acetabuli. A protusio acetabuli can occur when the floor of the acetabulum is destroyed, e.g. inflammatory arthritis or fractured, e.g. central fracture dislocation of the hip (Fig. 9.12).

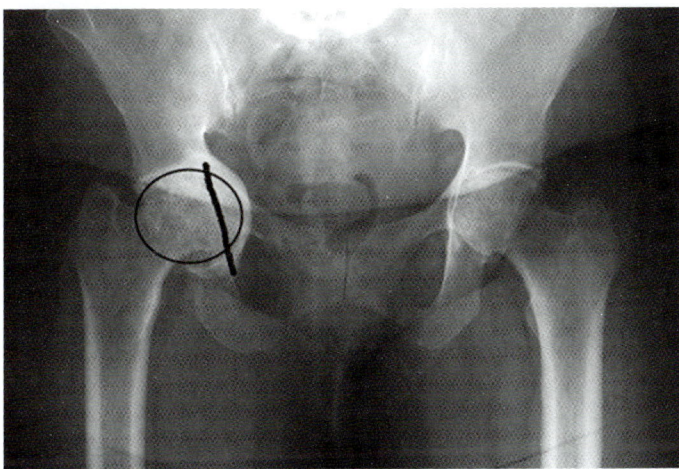

Fig. 9.12: Protusio acetabuli

Acetabular Version

In vertical anatomical position of the pelvis, the acetabulum cavity is not oriented purely to the lateral side; it is oriented anterolaterally, i.e. acetabulum is anteverted. In a plain radiograph of the hip which is a single planar investigation, it is not possible to appreciate the exact anteversion of the acetabulum. An indirect evidence can be accessed from the X-ray to know whether the acetabulum is anteverted or retroverted. The anterior and the posterior parts of the acetabular rim create separate outlines on the X-ray. In a normally anteverted acetabulum, the outline of the anterior rim doesn't cross the outline of the posterior rim (Fig. 9.13A). In a retroverted acetabulum, these outlines (of anterior rim or posterior rim) cross (Fig. 9.13B).

Congruency

The convex outline of the femoral head is symmetrical and corresponds to the concavity of the acetabular cavity in all radiographic views. These run strictly parallel to each other in a symmetrical manner. If the symmetry is lost, the hip joint is called incongruous.

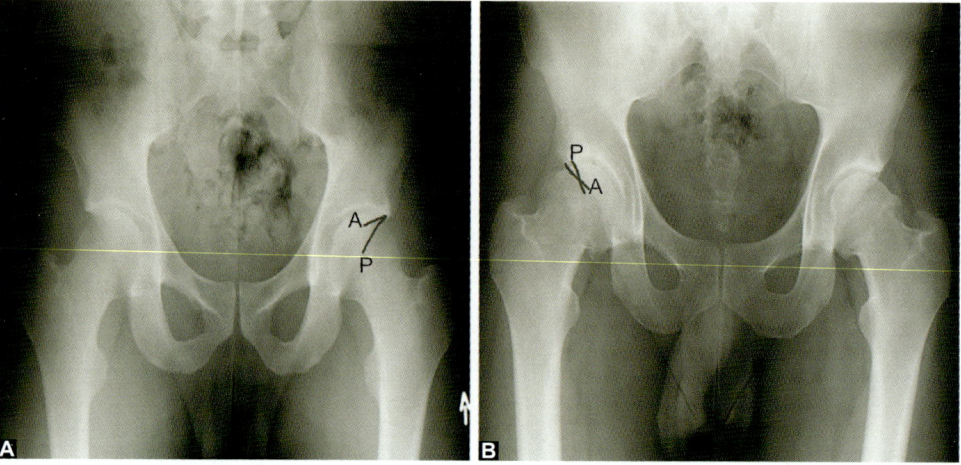

Fig. 9.13A and B: Acetabular version, as appearing in the AP radiograph: (A) Normal anteversion; (B) Retroversion with 'crossover' sign

HEAD–NECK CHARACTERISTICS INCLUDING OFFSET

- General characteristics
- Coxa magna
- Neck-shaft angle
- Head–neck offset
- Trabecular pattern

General Characteristics (Fig. 9.14)

Make a note of the general shape and outline of the head and the neck. The head may be irregular or destroyed like in an inflammatory arthritis. The density of the head should be noted—increased density indicates avascular necrosis. The extent and location of the avascular area should be noted.

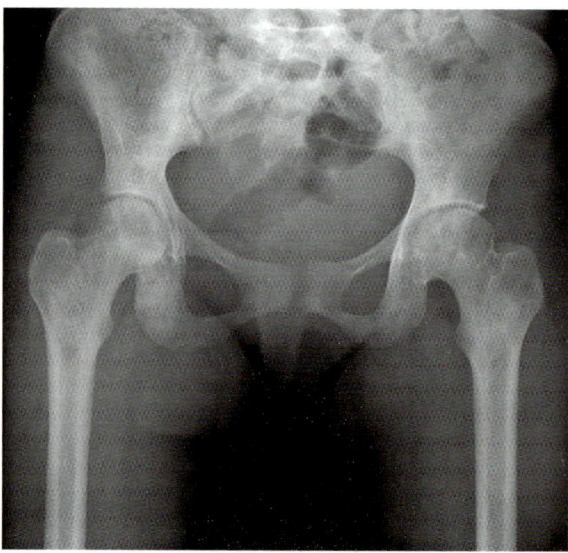

Fig. 9.14: Anteroposterior view of the normal hip

Coxa Magna

The head and the neck may become broad and short in cases of Perthes disease. This is called coxa magna (Fig. 9.15).

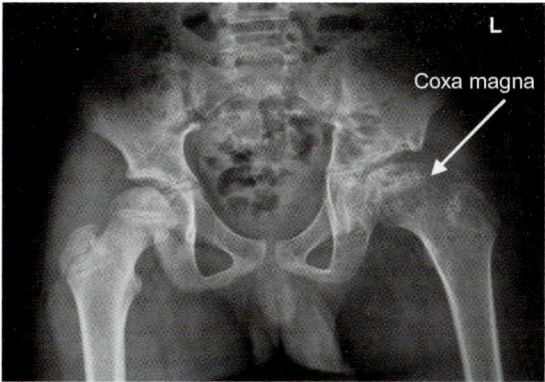

Fig. 9.15: Coxa magna

Neck-Shaft Angle (Fig. 9.16)

The angle between the central axes of the head and neck segments, and upper shaft makes an angle of 125 to 135° normally. The angle may decrease in some situations, like malunited trochanteric fracture; such a decreased neck-shaft angle is called coxa vara. On the other hand, in a few situations, the neck-shaft angle may be increased beyond 135°, e.g. congenital dysplasia of the hip. Such a condition is called coxa valga.

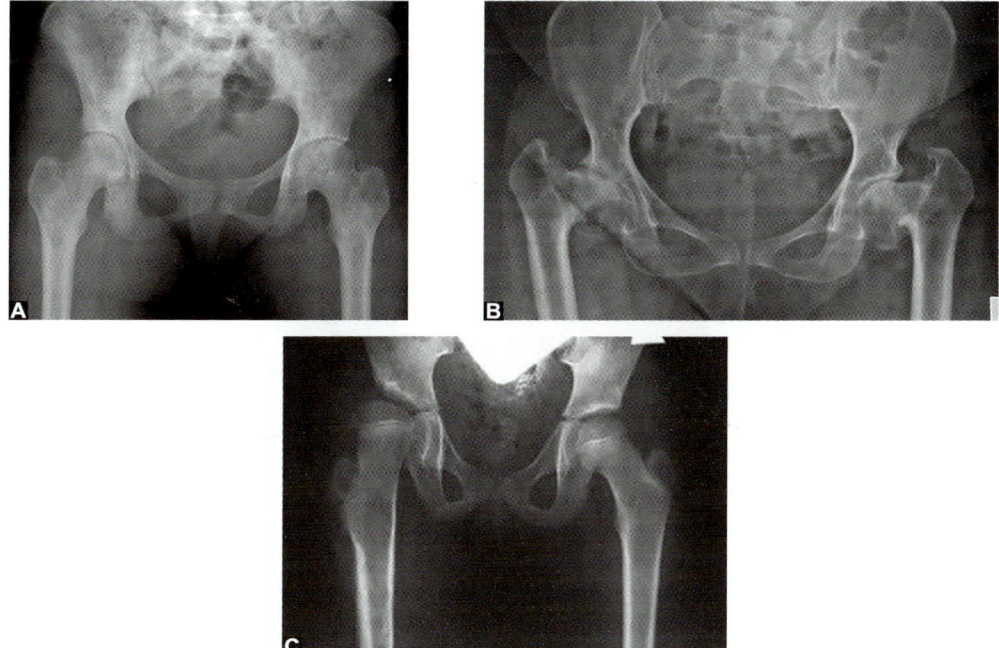

Fig. 9.16A to C: (A) Normal; (B) Coxa vara; (C) Coxa valga

Head–Neck Offset (Fig. 9.17)

Head–neck offset is a measure of the lateralization of the shaft of femur from the centre of the hip. On a plain radiograph of the hip, it is the distance between the centre of the head and tip of the trochanter. A normal offset is essential for optimal function of the abductors of the hip joint. If head and/or neck is destroyed, the offset will be decreased.

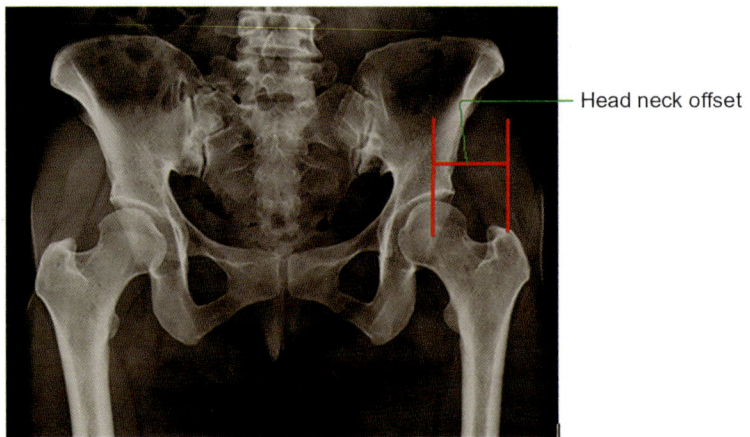

Fig. 9.17: Head–neck offset

Trabecular Pattern (Fig. 9.18)

Trabeculae in the upper end of the femur are arranged in well-defined groups:
- Principal compressive/medial compressive trabeculae
- Principal tensile trabeculae
- Secondary compressive/lateral compressive trabeculae
- Secondary tensile trabeculae
- Greater trochanteric trabeculae

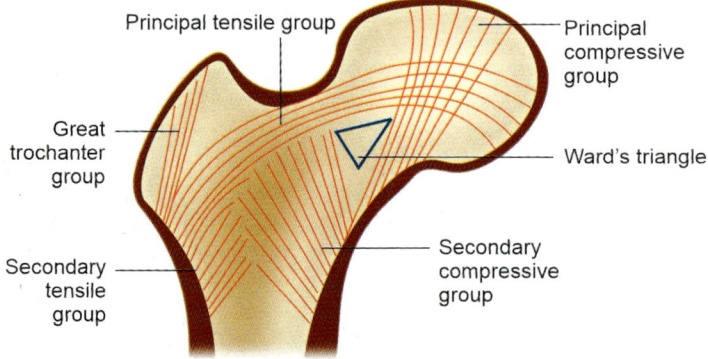

Fig. 9.18: Trochanteric pattern

These trabeculae have been laid down as per Wolff's law. In a good quality X-ray, they can be distinctly seen. After the onset of osteoporosis, they start disappear on the

X-ray, one by one. Depending upon their presence/absence, osteoporosis have been graded into different grades (Singh's index page no. 12)

RADIOGRAPHIC FINDINGS IN DIFFERENT HIP DISEASES

Common hip conditions:
- Neglected DDH
- Perthes disease
- Infantile coxa vara
- Old septic arthritis hip
- SCFE (slipped capital femoral epiphysis)
- Tuberculosis of hip
- Inflammatory arthritis of the hip joint—rheumatoid arthritis
- Bony ankylosis (in ankylosing spondylitis)
- Rickets and osteomalacia
- Femoral neck fracture
- Trochanteric fracture
- Dislocation of hip
- Osteoarthritis
- Tumours

Neglected DDH (Fig. 9.19)

It is not rare to find neglected DDH patients in our country. X-ray findings in these cases would be as follows:
- Congruency is partially/completely lost—head of the femur is obviously sub-luxated/dislocated, i.e. it is lying outside the quadrants found by Perkin's and Hilgenreiner's lines.
- Shenton line is broken.
- The dislocated head is likely to occupy a false acetabulum, superior to the original acetabulum.
- The original acetabulum is shallow and acetabular index is increased.
- Head of the femur may be deformed.
- Neck-shaft angle is likely to be increased (coxa valga).

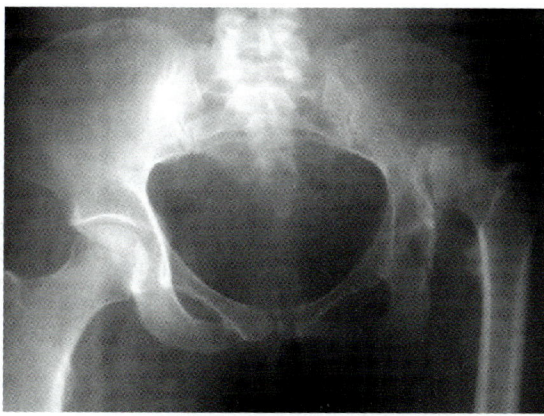

Fig. 9.19: Neglected DDH

Perthes Disease (Fig. 9.20)

A varying portion of the upper femur epiphysis shows increased density, because of the loss of blood supply. The extent and location of the avascular area varies. Complete collapse, flattening and fragmentation of the epiphysis occur in advanced cases. Once the collapse occurs, the head of the femur moves towards the superior side of the acetabulum and Shenton line would be broken. Lateral subluxation of the capital femoral epiphysis and resultant loss of congruity may be seen. Head and neck may become broad—coxa magna. Acetabular margin would be irregular, once the head is deformed. The severity of the disease is classified radiologically by two common systems—Catterall classification and Herring's lateral pillar classification (Tables 9.4 and 9.5).

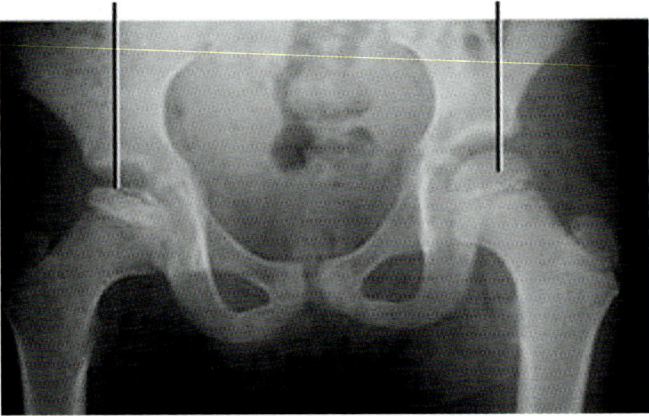

Fig. 9.20: Perthes disease

Table 9.4: Herring's lateral pillar classification		
Group A	Lateral pillar maintains full height without any density changes	
Group B	Maintains >50% height	
B/C border	Lateral pillar is narrowed (2–3 mm) or poorly ossified with approximately 50% height	

Contd.

Table 9.4: Herring's lateral pillar classification (*Contd.*)		
Group C	Less than 50% of lateral pillar height is maintained	

Table 9.5: Catterall classification		
Group 1	Involvement of the anterior epiphysis only	
Group 2	Involvement of the anterior epiphysis with a central sequestrum	
Group 3	Only a small part of the epiphysis is not involved	
Group 4	Total head involvement	

Infantile Coxa Vara

Radiological characteristics include:
- Decreased neck-shaft angle
- Small and flat femoral head
- Vertical orientation of epiphyseal plate.

The above findings would be present in other causes of coxa vara also.

The characteristics feature of infantile coxa vara is an abnormal triangular bony fragment, lying inferolateral to the epiphyseal plate and contained in an inverted Y-shape lucency (Fig. 9.21).

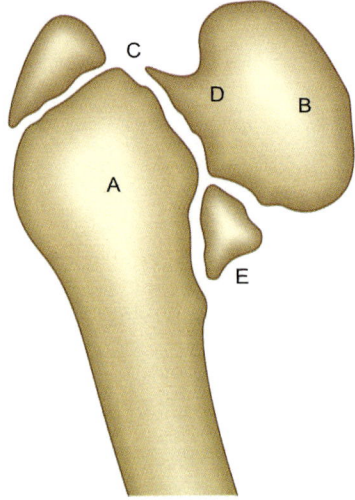

Fig. 9.21: Infantile coxa vara

Old Septic Arthritis Hip (Fig. 9.22)

Destruction of the upper femoral capital epiphysis, partial or complete, is evident. There may infact be complete absence of femoral head. Because of the destruction of the head, it gives an erroneous impression of increased joint space. Limb is obviously

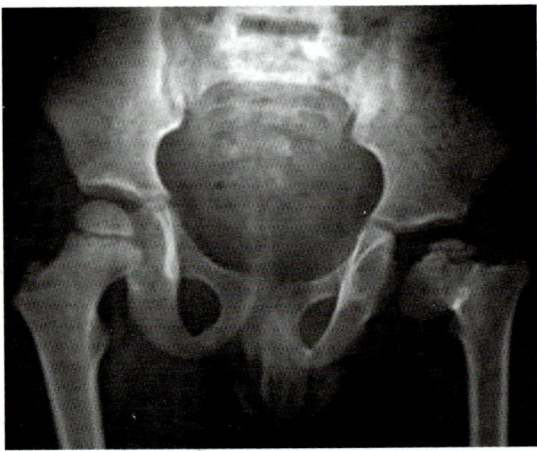

Fig. 9.22: Old septic arthritis hip

short—lesser trochanter on the same side is at a higher level. Shenton line is broken. In long-standing cases, the acetabulum index would be increased (i.e. acetabulum would be more vertical) and it will be shallow. The margins of acetabulum may be irregular, and sclerosed because of healed infection.

Slipped Capital Femoral Epiphysis (SCFE) (Fig. 9.23)

In the initial stages, the findings may be very subtle in AP view (Fig. 9.23A). The AP view may look normal on a cursory look. However, on drawing the Klein's line, it will be found that it does not intersect the capital epiphysis and the epiphysis lies below this line on the affected side. The lateral films will clinch the diagnosis and show the inferomedial slip of the epiphysis (Fig. 9.23B). Over a period of time, coxa vara deformity would be noticed. In late cases, there may be chondrolysis and destruction of the epiphysis.

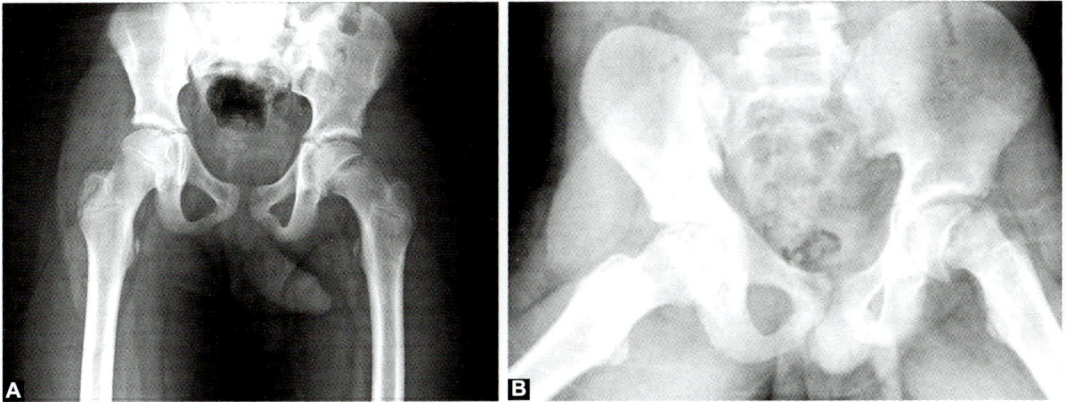

Fig. 9.23A and B: SCFE (slipped capital femoral epiphysis): (A) AP view; (B) Frog leg lateral view

Tuberculosis of Hip (Fig. 9.24)

It is not uncommon in India and infact is one of the main differential diagnoses of any chronic hip ailment in this country. It causes varying degree of destruction of acetabulum as well as the head of the femur.

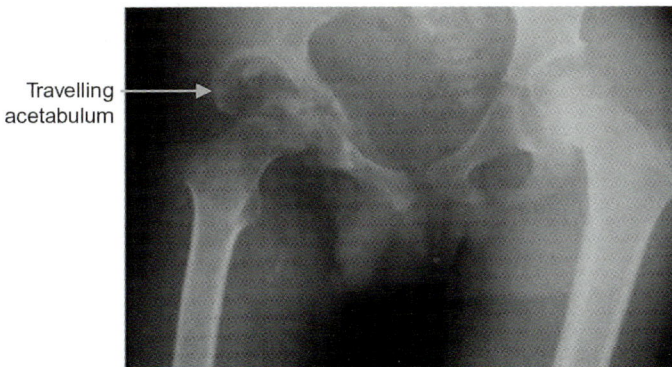

Fig. 9.24: Tuberculosis of hip

Dr. Shanmugasundaram TK in 1983 has identified 6 different types of radiological pictures of tuberculosis hip (Figs 9.25 and 9.26).

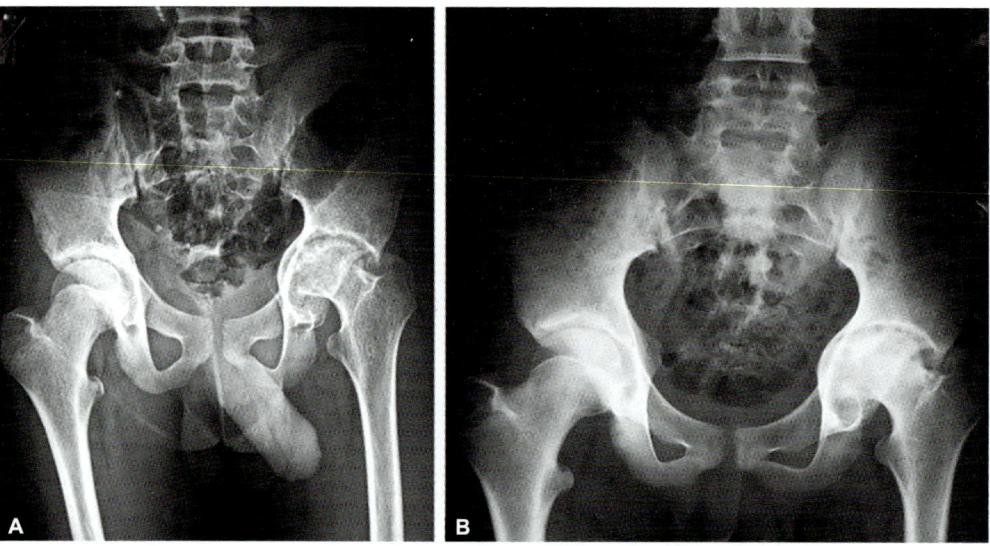

Fig. 9.25A and B: Tuberculsis of the hip type-5—protusio acetabuli: (A) Active; (B) Heeled

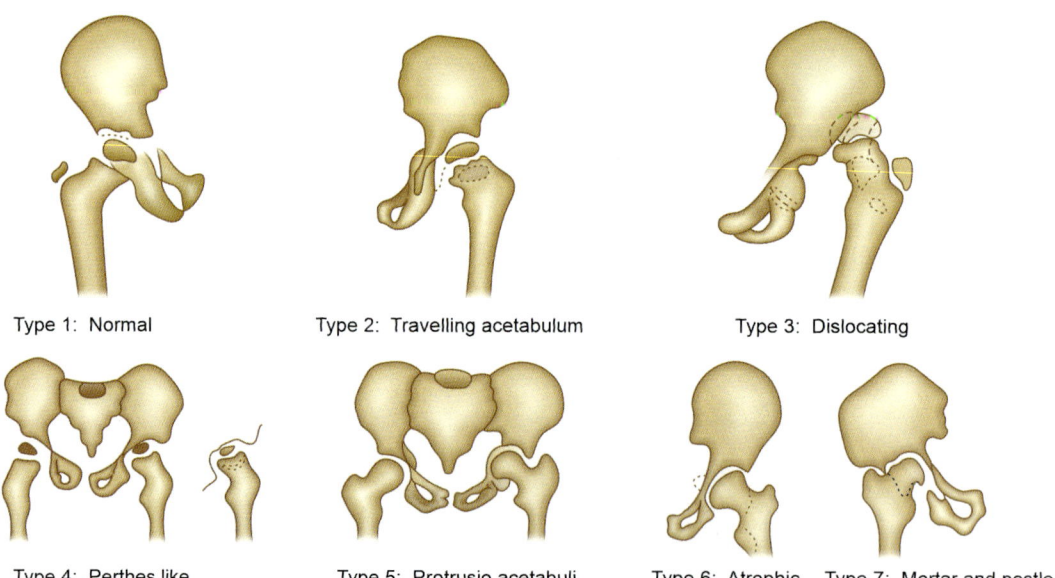

Fig. 9.26: Dr. Shanmugasundaram types of tuberculosis of hip

- **Type 1: Normal**
- **Type 2: Travelling acetabulum**: Destruction of the superior lateral wall and adjacent bone gives the impression that acetabulum has become larger and is taking a new position, since the destroyed part is in continuity with the apparently intact lower part of acetabulum.

- **Type 3: Dislocating**: In cases of destruction of superolateral part of acetabulum, along with flexor adductor spasm, the head of the femur starts dislocating in a posterior and superior direction.
- **Type 4: Perthes like**: Avascular necrosis of the femoral epiphysis due to compromised blood supply causes flattened and dense capital epiphysis.
- **Type 5: Prutusio acetabuli:** Destruction of the medial wall of acetabulum causes the head to shift inside the pelvis.
- **Types 6 and 7: Atrophic and mortar and pestle**: Decreased growth of various epiphyses because of compromised blood supply.

However, these distinct types may not be observed everytime and it is not unusual to find a combination of these, with a varied radiological appearance. Other findings may include coxa magna (enlargement of head and the neck), coxa breva (decrease in the dimensions of head of the femur), coxa valga and coxa vara. Outline of the acetabulum may be irregular and destroyed. Diffused osteoporosis around the affected hip joint is present in acute cases.

Inflammatory Arthritis of the Hip Joint—Rheumatoid Arthritis

Various types of inflammatory non-infective arthritis give rise to similar picture. The commonest arthritis in this class is rheumatoid arthritis. The X-ray will depend upon the severity and duration of the illness. There is destruction and irregularity of the joint margins of acetabulum, as well as the head of the femur, loss of the joint space, protusio acetabuli with break in the Shenton's line. Soft tissue oedema and swelling may be appreciable on the X-ray. The changes are likely to be present on both the sides.

Bony Ankylosis (in Ankylosing Spondylitis)

In ankylosing spondylitis, one may find bony ankylosis across the affected hip joint, in late stages. Other features on the X-ray will give clues to the diagnosis of ankylosing spondylitis like calcification of the ligaments in the vicinity of sacroiliac joint (sacrotuberous) and longitudinal ligaments in the lower part of the lumbosacral spine, visible in the X-ray taken for pelvis (Fig. 9.27).

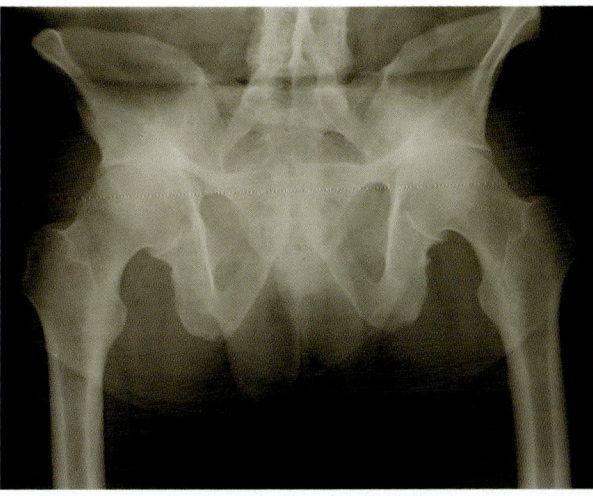

Fig. 9.27: Bony ankylosis (in ankylosing spondylitis)

The sacroiliac joints may be fused because of the disease.

In India, bony ankylosis of the hip may be seen in other conditions like cases of healed tuberculosis of the hip, particularly with super added pyogenic infection following a draining sinus. Septic arthritis of the hip in adults, which can cause bony ankylosis, is rarely seen, unless there is an underline cause, particularly when there is compromised immunity, e.g. HIV infection, prolonged steroid intake, uncontrolled diabetes, etc. Septic arthritis of the hip at younger age, in infancy and early childhood, is common, but it would result in dissolution of cartilaginous head and a resultant unstable joint, rather than an ankylosed joint.

Rickets and Osteomalacia

These two conditions follow the failure of mineralization of the osteoid due to disturbance of vitamin D metabolism. Rickets occurs before epiphyseal closure, while osteomalacia occurs after epiphyseal closure. There is unavailability of bioactive form of vitamin D, which could follow many possible causes like low nutritional intake, poor absorption from GI tract, or failure to convert to bioactive form due to renal or/ and liver disease.

In rickets, which occurs in childhood, since the epiphyseal plate is open, there is collection of the unmineralized osteoid in the epiphyseal plate. The epiphyseal plate of the growing ends of the bone particularly around knee and wrist are widened. The epiphyseal plate at the upper end of the femur will also be widened and there is irregularity and fuzziness of its borders. Coxa vara may occur. The bones in the neighbourhood show osteoporosis (Fig. 9.28).

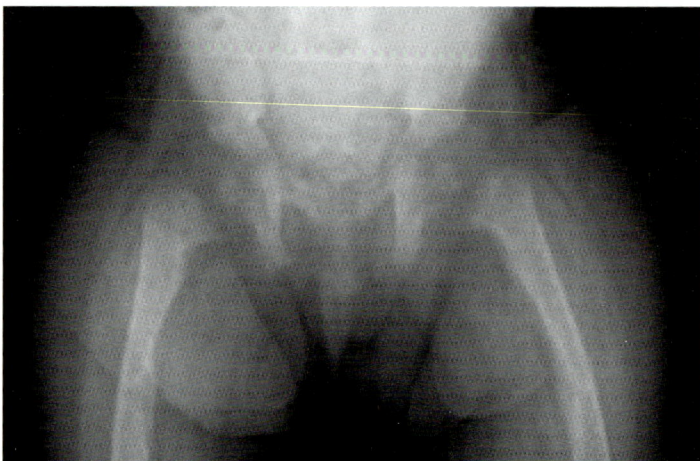

Fig. 9.28: Rickets with coxa vara and other manifestations

In osteomalacia, which occurs when the growth is over and the epiphyseal plate is closed, there will be other manifestations of unmineralized osteoid. Typically Looser's zones are seen which are poorly healed stress fractures, since there is failure of mineralization. These are visible on X-ray as linear lucencies, lying perpendicular to the cortex. These Looser's zones are characteristically seen in medial cortex of the neck of the femur, pubic and ischial rami, in the X-ray of pelvis with both hips. These are seen in ribs and scapulae also.

Fracture Neck of the Femur

It is a common fracture in old age. The X-ray picture can be described as per various classifications available.

1. **Anatomical classification:** As per the location of the fracture line:
   a. Subcapital
   b. Transcervical
   c. Basicervical

   Neck of the femur is an intracapsular fracture except basicervical, which can be partially extracapsular.

2. **Garden classification:** It describes the extent of fracture, as well as, relative orientation of disrupted trabeculae in proximal and distal fragments (Fig. 9.29 and Table 9.6).

Table 9.6: Garden staging		
Type	*Description*	*Non-displaced or displaced*
I	✘ Valgus impacted incomplete fracture ✘ The trabeculae in the proximal and distal fragments form an angle, towards superior side	Non-displaced
II	✘ Complete, non-displaced fracture ✘ Trabeculae in proximal and distal fragments are in line	Non-displaced
III	✘ Complete fracture, partial displacement ✘ Trabeculae in distal and proximal fragments form an angle, towards inferior side	Displaced
IV	✘ Complete fracture, complete displacement ✘ Trabeculae in proximal and distal fragments are discontinuous but parallel	Displaced

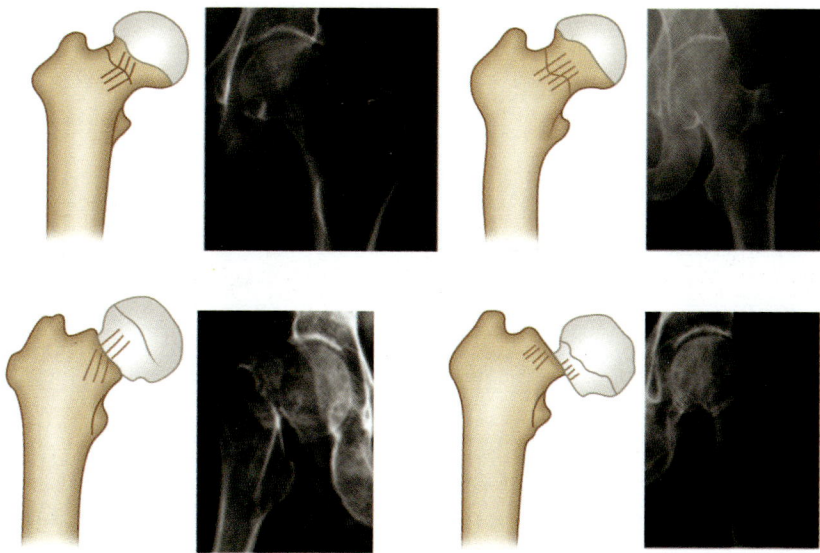

Fig. 9.29: Garden staging

3. **Pauwels classification:** This classification describes the angle of the fracture line to the horizontal. As the angle becomes more vertical, shearing force is increased. Three grades have been described in Table 9.7.

Table 9.7: Pauwels classification	
Grade 1	Less than 30° from horizontal
Grade 2	30–50° from horizontal
Grade 3	More than 50° from horizontal

Trochanteric Fracture

Trochanteric fractures occur commonly in the elderly following a minor fall. They can occur at a younger age also, where a significant force is required to break the trochanteric area. The classification, which is based on extent of the injury (area involved, comminution, orientation of fracture lines) and the likely prognosis is the one described by Boyd and Griffin (Fig. 9.30). It has four different types as follows:
- Type I: Stable two part
- Type II: Unstable comminuted
- Type III: Unstable reverse oblique
- Type IV: Intertrochanteric–subtrochanteric with two planes of fracture

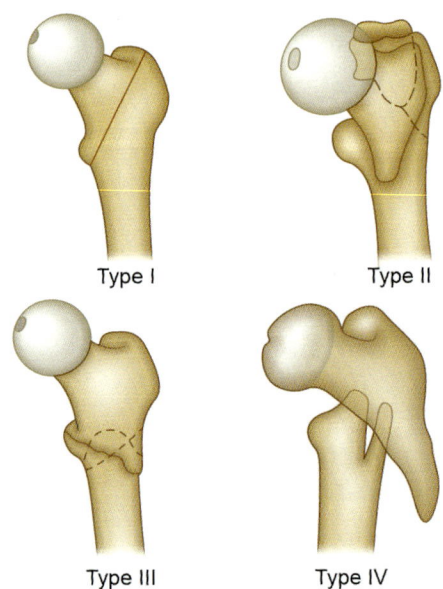

Type I   Type II

Type III   Type IV

Fig. 9.30: Boyd and Griffin classification (1949).[Type 1 is stable and rest are unstable.]

Dislocation of Hip

There is an obvious disruption of the head and acetabular articulation. Shenton's line is broken. Depending upon the direction, the types of hip dislocation have been described:
1. Posterior
2. Anterior
3. Inferior
4. Central

The commonest type is posterior dislocation in which the femur can be seen to be adducted in the X-ray. Look specifically for any associated fracture. In posterior dislocation of the hip, the commonest associated fracture is the fracture of the posterior wall of the acetabulum.

Osteoarthritis (Fig. 9.31)

The radiographic hallmark of osteoarthritis is joint space narrowing. This narrowing is associated with subchondral sclerosis, marginal osteophytes, cyst formation, and later superolateral subluxation of the femoral head. Once subluxation starts occurring, Shenton's line will be broken. Altered weight bearing due to traumatic injury or congenital anomalies may predispose to early development of osteoarthritis. Primary osteoarthritis of the hip is rare in our country though quite prevalent in western societies. In India and other Asian countries, osteoarthritis of the hip is mostly secondary to a traumatic damage or a congenital anomaly which predisposes to secondary osteoarthritic changes.

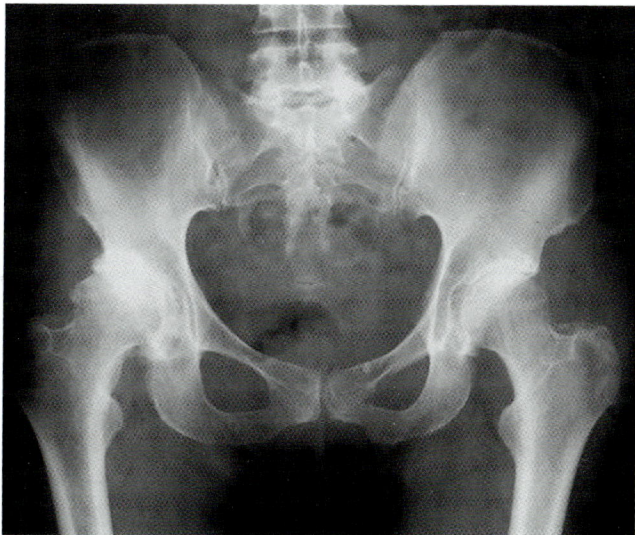

Fig. 9.31: Osteoarthritis of right hip

Tumours

The most common primary malignant tumour of pelvic area is chondrosarcoma. It is usually a well-demarcated tumour and shows increased areas of radiodensity. The other pelvic tumour which could be seen in a radiograph of pelvis with both hips is chordoma of the sacrum. It appears as an osteolytic mass involving the sacrum. Another common sacral tumour is giant cell tumour.

The tumours which can per se involve upper end of the femur include osteoid osteoma, osteochondroma, giant cell tumour of the head and the neck and rarely osteosarcoma arising from the upper metaphyseal area of femur. It is beyond the scope of this book to describe individual tumours.

Pelvis is a common site for metastatic bone tumours—particularly from prostatic carcinoma in males and cervical malignancy in females.

Index